BIKE FIT

2ND EDITION

BIKE FIT

OPTIMISE YOUR BIKE POSITION FOR HIGH PERFORMANCE AND INJURY AVOIDANCE

PHIL BURT

BLOOMSBURY SPORT

LONDON · OXFORD · NEW YORK · NEW DELHI · SYDNEY

I dedicate this book to
my wonderful wife Claire and
children Noah and Esme without
whose support this book would
have been impossible to write. Also, to
Nik Cook, who makes anyone's words better!

BLOOMSBURY SPORT
Bloomsbury Publishing Plc
50 Bedford Square, London,
WC1B 3DP, UK
29 Earlsfort Terrace, Dublin 2, Ireland

BLOOMSBURY, BLOOMSBURY SPORT
and the Diana logo are trademarks of
Bloomsbury Publishing Plc

First published in Great Britain 2014
This edition published 2022

Copyright © Phil Burt, 2022
Illustrations © XAB Design, with
the exception of the following:
pp. 25 and 26 © Shutterstock;
p. 119 © Getty Images 2022

Studio photography by Grant
Pritchard, Cycling photography
© Getty Images with the exception
of the following: p 12 © Endura;
pp. 120, 123 LH, p. 144 © Shutterstock;
pp. 154, 156, 158 and 160–161 © Zwift

Phil Burt has asserted his
right under the Copyright,
Designs and Patents Act, 1988, to
be identified as Author of this work.

For legal purposes the
Acknowledgements on page 207
constitute an extension of this
copyright page.

A catalogue record for this book
is available from the British Library.

Library of Congress Cataloguing-in-
Publication data has been applied for.

ISBN: 978-1-4729-9018-1
eBook: 978-1-4729-9011-2

10 9 8 7 6 5 4 3 2 1

Printed and bound in China by Toppan
Leefung Printing

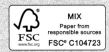

To find out more about our authors
and books visit www.bloomsbury.com
and sign up for our newsletters.

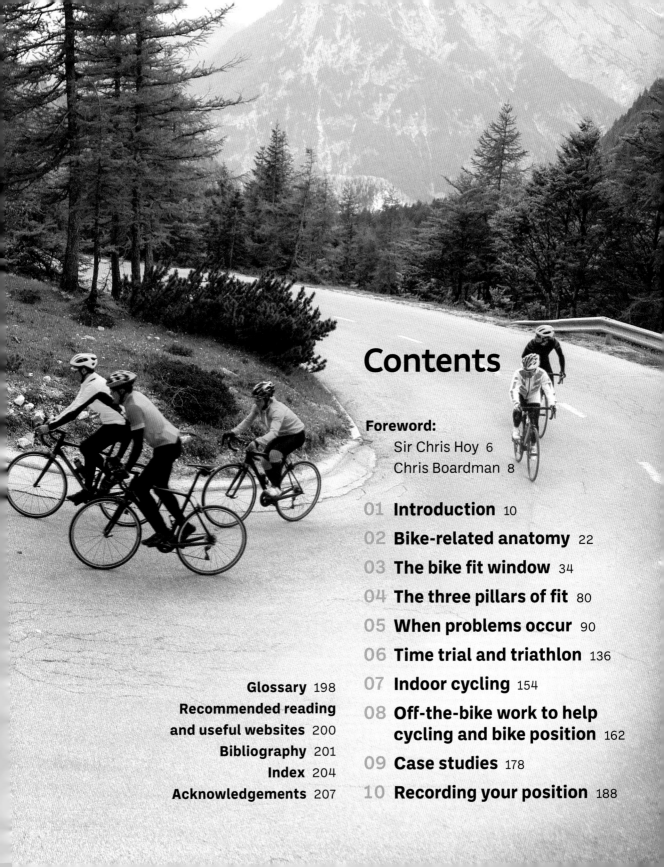

Contents

Foreword:
Sir Chris Hoy

I love seeing so many people out on bikes, but few things frustrate me more than seeing someone riding a machine that is poorly set up.

When I speak to new cyclists, it is striking how often they complain of a sore bum, or a bad back or an injured knee. They've tried cycling, they say, but find it painful, uncomfortable or both – and therefore not very enjoyable.

I cannot understand it, because I love riding my bike and, unless repeating flat-out efforts on the track in training, do find it enjoyable. But I would say that 99 times out of 100 they are in pain not because the saddle is too hard or that riding a bike is too strenuous. It is because the bike has not been set up correctly.

Similarly, when people ask me for advice about riding a charity event or sportive, perhaps for the first time, they are often looking for training tips.

They want to know what distances to ride and how often. Before you worry about that, I say, make sure your position is right.

Riding a bike with the wrong position is a bit like trying to run in somebody else's shoes. I arrived at the 'right' position through lots of trial and error, but also with the help of some expert advice, from coaches and experienced riders.

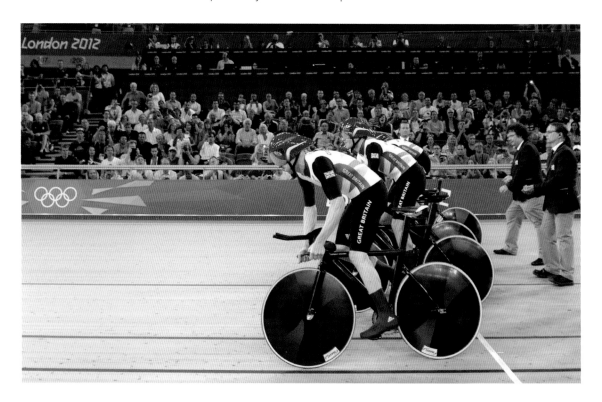

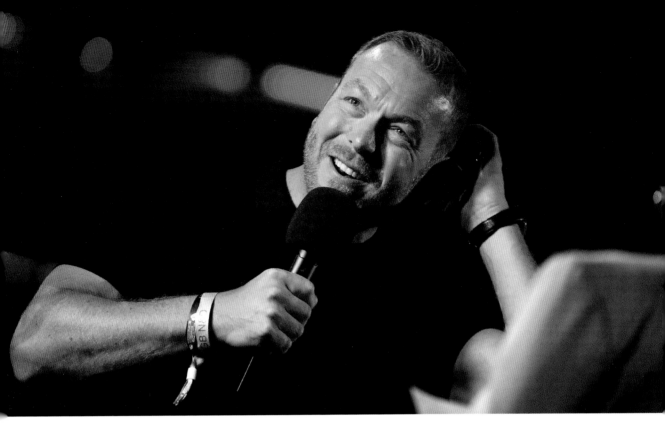

I ended up riding in the same position for 15 years and now I don't need a tape-measure to tell me if the three points of contact – bottom, hands and feet – are correct for me. I can do it on feel. I can hop on a bike and tell you if the saddle is half a centimetre too high or too low.

As a full-time cyclist you become really attuned to your position and very sensitive to any changes. I remember in the first part of the 2003 season my saddle height was slightly out – it was a tiny bit too high. The change was marginal, but it gave me knee problems almost immediately.

The person who helped me overcome such injuries for almost a decade was Phil Burt. I've worked with numerous physiotherapists, but leading up to the Beijing and London Olympic Games I spent as much time talking to and seeking advice from Phil as from my coaches.

I can honestly say that he did as much as anyone to keep me in one piece, especially in the build-up to London when at times my 36-year-old body seemed to be giving up on me. As well as being a really nice bloke, he is also a very big guy so he has always been able to manipulate my back better than most.

But it is on the subject of bike position that Phil has become an expert. I perhaps wouldn't have needed as much trial and error over 20 years ago if I had known Phil then.

It is great that he has now collected his knowledge in this book. My advice to any cyclist, new or old, has always been to seek expert advice from experienced cyclists, coaches or physios, or from a reputable bike shop. But there is also another option – to consult Phil's book.

I hope it means that when I'm out on my own bike, passing other cyclists – or, now that I have retired, being passed by them – I can admire others' positions on their bikes, rather than regretting the fact that they could be getting so much more enjoyment from their cycling – and avoiding injury – if only their saddle was the right height!

As I'm sure everyone can appreciate, it is so much more comfortable, efficient and fun to be running in your own shoes.

Chris Hoy

Foreword:
Chris Boardman

I am a spreadsheet kind of guy. I love understanding things, finding formulas and efficiency gains, so you'd think that bike fitting and position-finding would be right up my street.

It's probably not surprising, then, that together with my coach Peter Keen, a well-respected, even world-renowned sports scientist, I did indeed study the world of position efficiency while I was a professional cyclist for the best part of a decade. Because the nature of my job saw me ride events from four minutes to three weeks in duration, we explored and experimented in many different areas: climbing, long-distance riding, extreme track pursuit and, of course, time trialling.

For early work on time trial and track racing posture, we retreated to Peter's garage where, with the help of a full-length mirror and an ergometer (which measures how much work muscles do), we learned just how unknowingly closed-minded we actually were when it came to the topic of positions.

The ergometer allowed us almost infinite movement in any plane and the ability to consider geometry completely free of standard bicycle parts. In fact, apart from having a saddle, pedals and some handlebars, the contraption didn't even look like a bicycle, which would prove to be a huge breakthrough.

On one occasion, we had embarked on a session to investigate aerodynamic positions. We used the full-length mirror set out in front to monitor my silhouette (or frontal area) with the goal of minimising this while I monitored mechanical efficiency with each change we made. Due to the strange shape of the ergometer, we explored on feel, without measuring until we arrived at something we felt looked promising and that I felt I could maintain for the duration of the event we were training for. Only then did we measure things and find just what it all translated to in terms of frame sizes and stem lengths, our usual stock in trade. Had we been on standard and recognisable equipment, our concept of what a

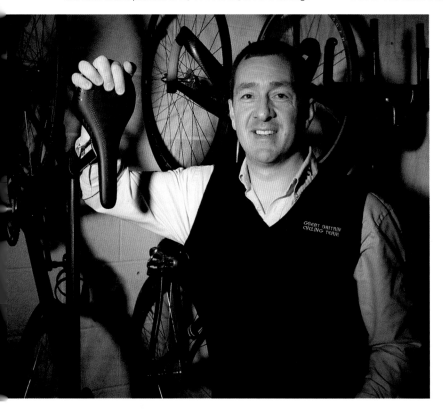

bike rider could do would have prevented us from ever exploring, and subsequently finding, the position we had now settled upon. From that moment on, we never measured during a positional session, not until after we had finished evaluating ideas, lest our own prejudices encouraged us to ignore more important data.

We carried this philosophy on when studying climbing positions too. This time our goal was to find an efficient and sustainable stance in which to tackle the mountain passes of the Tour de France. For this we pioneered the use of treadmills, first to explore, record and change positions in the lab (at Brighton University) and then to reinforce muscular learning with long stints of many hours' climbing under heat lamps to simulate the conditions of the great race.

No matter what type of riding you want to optimise your position for, the number of factors to be considered is enormous: personal sensitivity to small adjustments, individual body shape, individual muscularity, the type of bike being used, the type of riding you will do, how long you will typically be riding for, clothing, shoes and

so on. All of these things and much more influence the overall 'positional package'.

You will notice the term 'feel' crops up repeatedly in the above narrative and there is a reason for that. In all the time we explored the intricacies of bicycle positioning, we never found the magic formula. Indeed, I am now thoroughly convinced that there isn't a single recipe and never will be. However, what I do think is emerging – and evidence is in these pages – are solid procedures for coming to educated conclusions and consistently acceptable solutions for a wide variety of riding needs.

Phil Burt has probably spent more time looking at these issues with more of the world's top athletes and across more disciplines than any other person on the planet.

So if you believe, as I do, that positioning will always be a blend of good science and good judgement, I think you can feel confident that both can be found between the covers of this book.

Chris Boardman

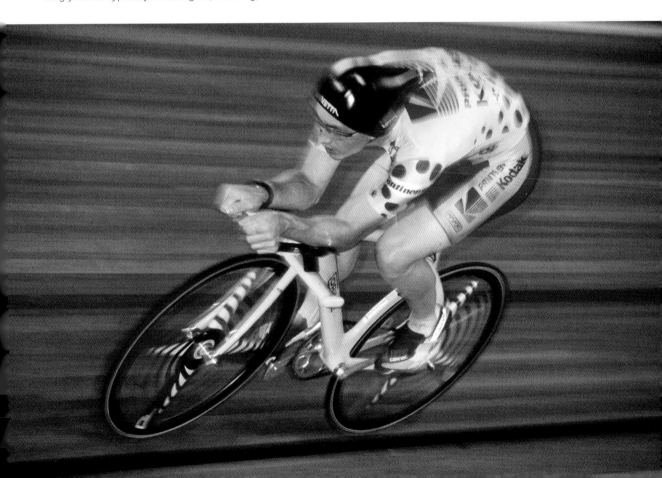

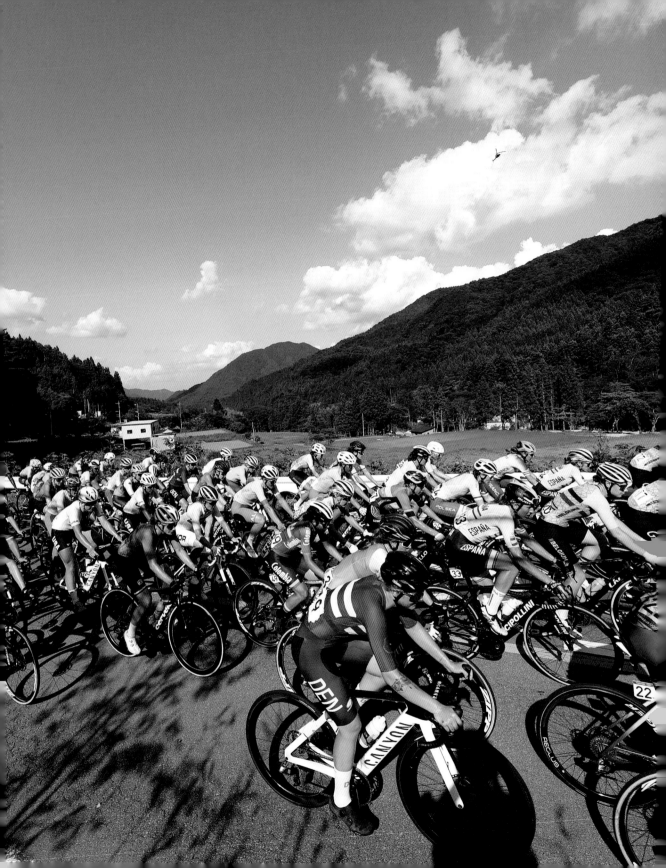

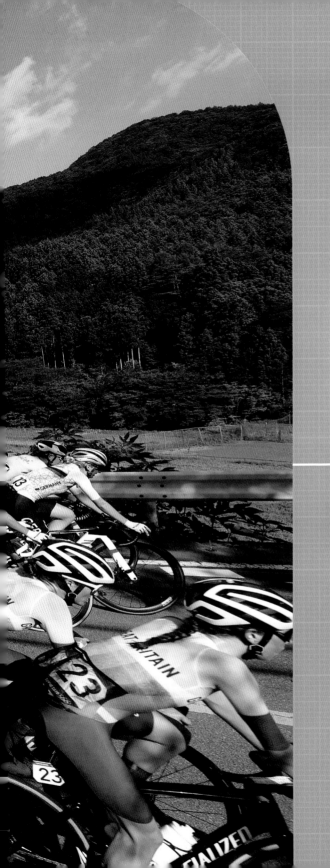

01

Introduction

Introduction

The concept of finding one perfect position on a bike is, in my opinion, fundamentally flawed as that position, no matter whether you're a Grand Tour contender, Olympic champion or weekend warrior sportive rider, is impacted by multiple variables.

It will also be constantly evolving. Whether it's the type of riding you're doing (your position will be very different on a time trial bike compared to a mountain bike), the impact of off-the-bike factors (positives such as improvements in mobility or negatives such as injury) or even the time of year (you might prefer a more relaxed position for winter training than for summer racing), how you set up your bike should be a journey that will go on for as long as you keep riding your bike. In the same way, my education as a bike fitter is ongoing and I genuinely learn something from every rider I work with.

My bike-fitting journey

It all started when I graduated with a degree in pharmacology and quickly realised I didn't want to work in a lab or as a drugs salesman. I wanted to be hands-on and face to face with the people I was helping and so opted for physiotherapy at Manchester. While I was studying I did some work with Manchester Rugby Club, before spending time in Australia, New Zealand and then running a ski clinic in Courchevel. Coming back to the UK, I happened to be in the right

Phil in the bike fit studio

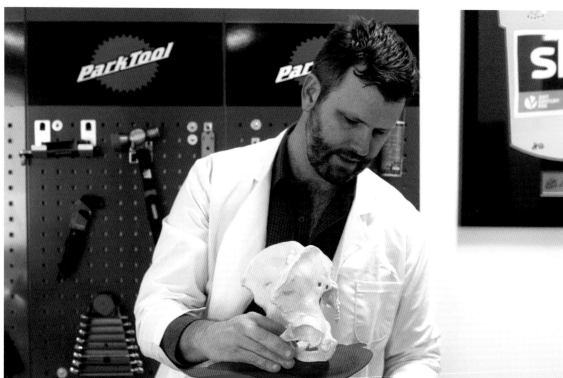

place at the right time and landed a job at Sale Sharks. During my three years at the club we were arguably the dominant force in English club rugby and in my last season there, in 2006, we won the Premiership title.

I then applied for a job via the English Institute of Sport and ended up in a role that was split between cycling and water polo. This then morphed into a full-time position with British Cycling and, from having been primarily concerned with soft tissue trauma from collisions in rugby, I was now faced with the complex interaction between riders and their bikes. It was a steep learning curve. At that point I looked for a book on the subject, but it didn't exist. I had to train in bike fitting with CycleFit in London (and I ended up writing the book I'd been looking for myself). In hindsight, though, that broad sporting background, whether rugby, squash, skiing or water polo, has proved invaluable now I'm working with the wider cycling population, as many of the riders I deal with have either played or still play another sport along with riding their bike.

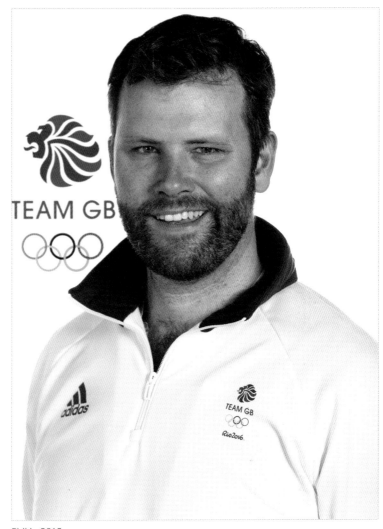

Phil in 2012

It was an incredibly exciting time to be involved with British Cycling and the whole story of the Medal Factory and the Secret Squirrel Club has been well documented. It all started with Peter Keen and then was finessed by the likes of Chris Boardman, Steve Peters and, of course, Dave Brailsford. The simple premise was that medals equal more funding, which leads to improvements, which means more medals and so the virtuous circle goes on. The most controllable medals to target were in the timed events on the track, where luck and external factors can be largely removed and so those were what we focused on. In 2006, Dave Brailsford made the incredibly gutsy call to give half of his budget to

Chris Boardman and simply told him to go away and make the best bikes, wheels and skin suits he possibly could. That was really the start of the whole 'marginal gains' approach, but the results we achieved at the 2008 Beijing Olympics were far from a marginal improvement, they were revolutionary.

This Olympic success gave Dave Brailsford the leverage to start approaching companies to sponsor a professional road team and Team Sky was born. He made the bold statement that we'd have a British Tour de France winner within five years and this definitely caused a few raised eyebrows. I was dispatched to investigate professional cycling and my simple conclusion was that it wasn't very professional and, if we approached it in the same way that we had the track, the gains were there to be made. Professional road cycling, especially on the Continent, was a sport still rooted in tradition and dogma, and it took Team Sky and its various subsequent manifestations to drag it kicking and screaming into a new era. A great example of this was that you never saw anyone warming down on a turbo trainer after a stage and we were laughed at when we started doing it. However, now it's the norm across the peloton.

Everything really came to fruition, both with Team Sky and British Cycling, in 2012 with Bradley Wiggins winning the Tour de France and our incredible success at a home Olympics. It really was amazing to be involved in and that summer is a period of my life that I'll never forget.

After 2012, my role within British Cycling evolved and, although still a hands-on physio, I was increasingly involved in equipment development and bike fit, and was part of the inner sanctum of the Secret Squirrel Club. Part of this was looking for the improvements we could make with a view to Rio in 2016 and a key area was saddle health, especially for our female riders. A significant number of our athletes were suffering saddle-related injuries, which was costing them training time, but it was being underreported by the riders, largely because of embarrassment, and therefore was being overlooked by coaches and support staff. Our investigations led to us question the UCI ruling on saddle tilt as we felt that their insistence on a level saddle was causing problems. We managed to convince them to change this rule, allowing for minus nine degrees of tilt, which significantly enhanced the comfort and health of all riders.

It was during this period that I wrote the first edition of this book. I remember at my first meeting with Bloomsbury I was asked why we should do this book, I answered that it didn't exist and their reply, which I admit threw me at the time, was to ask whether there was a reason for this! Fortunately, they trusted me that there was a market and a need for it, but getting it written was one of the hardest things I've ever done. I'm immensely proud of what I eventually produced and that book's DNA is at the heart of this one, but with hindsight and the broader experience I now have, there's a lot I missed.

Rio in 2016 was my third Olympics and again we managed to exceed our now stratospheric expectations. It was obvious, though, that the rest of the world, especially Australia, France, the Netherlands, USA and New Zealand, were closing the gap on us. I don't think this was down to any failings on our part, but was simply the combination of these nations putting similar models to ours in place, catching up in terms of technology and the fact that an extraordinary generation of riders were coming to the end of their careers.

For me, this was a natural end point for what had been an incredible time at British Cycling and I turned my attention to the wider cycling world, outside that elite performance bubble. Almost everything I did at British Cycling was geared towards winning medals, working with a tiny and very limited pool of riders, addressing their needs and developing equipment that would only benefit a handful of elite cyclists. I wanted to broaden my reach, my experience and my knowledge, and help the general cycling population.

It took me two years to actually take the plunge and, although the safety net of a part-time position at British Cycling was tempting, I knew I had to make a clean break to do what I wanted to do. Former colleagues, such as Steve Peters and Chris Boardman, encouraged me to join them outside the bubble in the real world, and my family were incredibly supportive and instrumental in my decision.

I set up my own bike fit studio at the Manchester Institute of Health and Performance and, suddenly, from having spent years dealing with an incredibly small sample group of clients, I had the full spectrum of the cycling population knocking on my door. On one hand that was really daunting and another steep learning curve, but on the other it was extremely liberating, as I was in control of the whole process with no coaches or directors to answer to. The variety was also really refreshing. I was dealing with triathletes, sportive riders who'd come to cycling late in life and even complete cycling novices – every fit was a learning experience and I felt I was making a real difference. Yes, it had been great helping to shave thousandths of a second off a lap of the velodrome in the quest for a gold medal, but getting a cyclist who's injured, in pain and suffering mentally from not being able to ride their bike, riding again is infinitely more satisfying. I was also freed from the Secret Squirrel Club and, rather than developing kit that would be rolled out for two weeks at the Olympics and never seen again, I was able to start working with companies to develop equipment that would be available to all riders. This brings me to now and my rationale for writing a second edition. As I've already alluded to, there were areas that I missed, but, more than that, both myself and the sport have evolved. I've now got a far wider experience and deeper understanding of cyclists across multiple disciplines, aspirations and backgrounds. We've seen more and more women entering the sport, the emergence of gravel cycling, the continued increase in the

popularity of triathlon – especially Ironman – and a huge surge in participation in indoor cycling and eRacing.

I'm more than aware that not all cyclists can afford a full professional bike fit, so my goal with this book is to give all riders the knowledge to begin their own bike fit journey to evolve their position to support their cycling needs. It's been immensely satisfying when I've had clients bring a copy of the first edition to a bike fit, asked me to sign it and told me that it's helped them to solve a problem. I'm confident that this new edition will reach even further, appeal to more riders, and help you to ride pain free and for years to come.

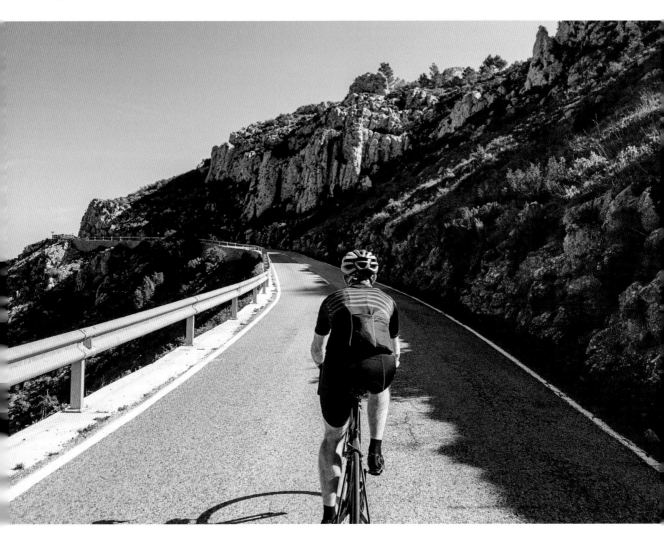

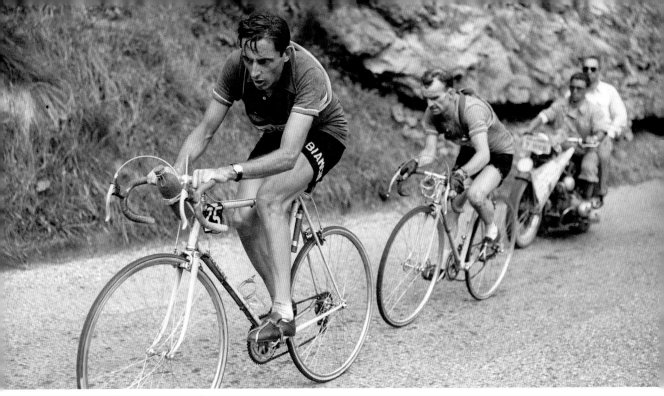

Fausto Coppi (*pictured on the left*)

Bike position: a brief history

Look at old pictures of racing cyclists and you can see how bike positions have changed and evolved. Fausto Coppi, the great Italian star of the 1940s and 50s, sat low with high handlebars – as did all his contemporaries. Jacques Anquetil, who came along in the late 1950s and dominated the Tour de France in the early 60s, still sat relatively low on the saddle (his legs weren't as extended as those of today's riders), but he looked to elongate his position; he was stretched across the bike, and looked quite aerodynamic. Others were naturally inspired to copy him. Change was often instigated by the best of any era.

Eddy Merckx, the greatest cyclist of all, followed Anquetil, and he was the catalyst for another change. He sat higher in the saddle, almost resembling a modern rider. Merckx was a micro-adjuster, always tweaking his saddle height and handlebars.

The first ever bike-fitting manual or book was published by CONI (the Italian Olympic Committee) in 1972. The Italians looked at a group of 20-year-old professional male cyclists who appeared to be successful and then set about describing the commonalities of their position on a bike. It was assumed that, because these riders were fast, their positions should be adopted by everyone. The resulting publication is often referred to as the 'Italian cycling bible' and it was treated as such for a long time. This meant that a lot of people were forced to adopt certain ways of sitting on their bikes. For example, it advocated a pigeon-toed pedalling style, with knees nearly touching the top tube. These days, we know that a large number of people simply cannot adapt to these styles of riding.

The Belgians were next on the scene. Like Italy, the country is a hotbed for cycling. But they kept position firmly in the x/y plane – viewing a rider's position from the side-on view only – and simply added a segmental approach to sizing. These were the first attempts to extrapolate someone's ideal bike size and position from a measure of leg inseam.

It was Cyrille Guimard, the legendary French directeur sportif behind Bernard Hinault and the Renault-Gitane team, who endorsed a formula that found popular appeal in the 1980s, not least because it was adopted by the American Tour de France winner,

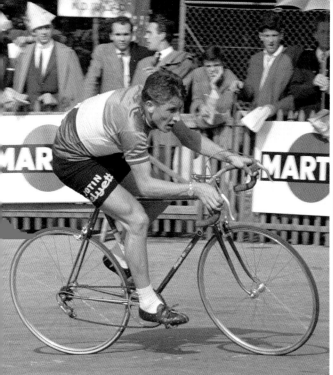

Jacques Anquetil

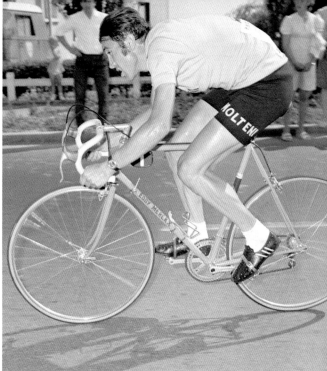

Eddy Merckx

Greg LeMond. This formula takes the rider's inseam length in centimetres and multiplies it by 0.883 to give the recommended saddle height (measured from the centre of the bottom bracket to the top of the saddle). The Guimard/LeMond formula makes some big assumptions – the main one being that all human beings grow in the same proportions. For example, it assumes that everyone's legs are in a specific ratio to the length of their backs and arms. Unfortunately, this just doesn't hold true in all cases. We all come in different shapes and sizes – and in different ratios of those shapes and sizes.

If you plotted the human race in terms of shape and size, for instance the relation of leg length to back length, you'd probably see a graph like the one on the following page.

Working out your bike size from an inseam measurement should work for those people in the middle third of the graph – the 'normal' ones – but for everybody else it will be out to varying degrees. For example, a long-legged person with a short back would be fine on the saddle, but be unable to comfortably reach the handlebars. Or someone with short legs and

a long back (such as Chris Boardman) would be fine with the reach, but end up sitting too high.

The situation becomes even more complicated when you consider the differences in people's degree of flexibility and control over their bodies. Simple extrapolations from chosen limb measurements can't account for this. I once rode Bradley Wiggins' bike back from a time trial at the Tour de Suisse. I am 6'4" and slightly taller than Brad. I could not believe how high he had his saddle. I could barely ride it and found it painful. I realised how much Bradley had adapted over the years of pursuiting to achieving a hamstring flexibility that allowed him to pedal in this super-efficient and powerful position.

Menwhile, another innovator, Andy Pruitt, has been working away at the Boulder Center for Sports Medicine in Colorado, USA. For the last 30 years he has been working in the field of cycling medicine and he was the first (and, to date, only) person to write a truly helpful medical guide for the cyclist. It remains one of the few books in print that takes the time to explore the concept of bike fit from a dynamic point of view, of the rider in motion as opposed to statically in position on the bike.

And it brought bike fitting into 3D with consideration to the frontal plane, that is, the rider's position as viewed from the front.

Dynamic bike fit gradually superseded the static fit, though it has taken a long time for the data-capture to be perfected and for the service to be accessible to non-professional cyclists. People can now turn up to clinics and laboratories to get their bike position assessed and modified to help them with performance, comfort or injury avoidance.

It was one of Andy Pruitt's co-workers who, in 2007, helped change the way we do bike fitting. Todd Carver helped develop and deliver one of the first 3D motion analysis systems that was easy to use (i.e. not research or laboratory based) specifically for cycling – the Retül system. This package of hardware and software could

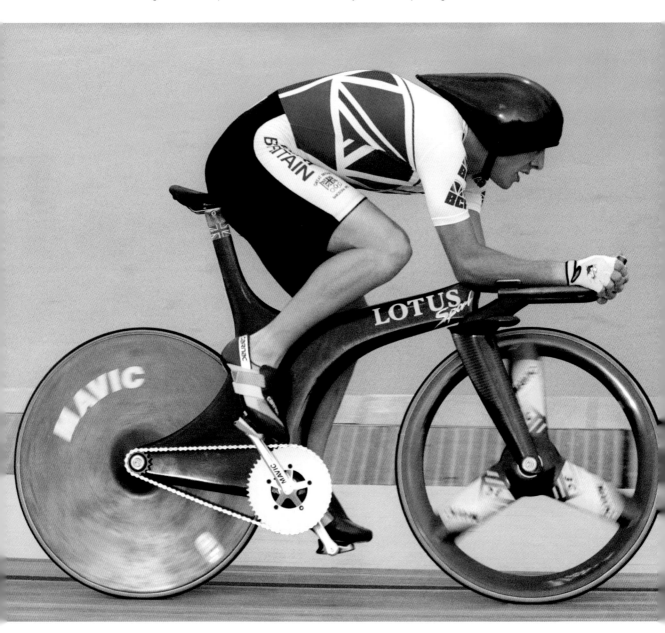

▶ Graph of normal distribution

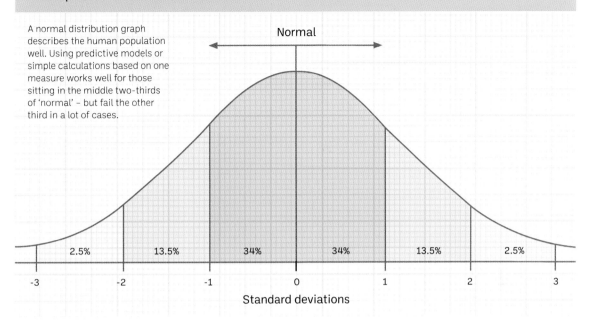

A normal distribution graph describes the human population well. Using predictive models or simple calculations based on one measure works well for those sitting in the middle two-thirds of 'normal' – but fail the other third in a lot of cases.

Normal

| 2.5% | 13.5% | 34% | 34% | 13.5% | 2.5% |

-3   -2   -1   0   1   2   3

Standard deviations

record not only biometric data but bike data as well, and do so within seconds. It changed the game for dynamic fit – today a cyclist can drop in to a good clinic, studio or shop and receive fitting advice using state of the art technology within hours rather than days.

Dynamic fit can be expensive – you could spend limitless amounts of money on these services. It is a great tool, but not necessarily the panacea. What the evolution of dynamic fit has created is a spectrum along which bike fit services can be plotted. The first methods

◀ A great example of a well-known cyclist the Guimard/LeMond method won't work for is Chris Boardman. The next time you see the great man on TV, take a few seconds to examine his overall composition. He has a very long back compared to his relatively short legs. This anomaly is probably what enabled him to adopt the incredibly low, flat-back aerodynamic position that helped to win Olympic Pursuit Gold and Tour de France Prologues. Chris would never have come to his position if he'd simply followed off the peg formulae.

of using static measurements of the rider and bike can maybe now be considered 'sizing' for a bike. The later dynamic methods, depending on their level of application, are more in line with this statement from the Medicine in Cycling group: 'A bike fit is the detailed process of evaluating the cyclist's physical and performance requirements and abilities and systematically adjusting the bike to meet the cyclist's goals and needs.'

So what does the recreational cyclist or the keen new sportive rider do when they can't find the solution to their positional issue, be it pain, injury, discomfort or underperformance?

You're unlikely to spend £300 on a bike fit if your bike only cost between £500 and £1,000. I'd like to think this book will bridge the gap between occasional cyclists and wealthier, top-end riders, and will provide the majority of today's cyclists with a handy guide to help you help yourselves. I aim to arm you with the information to make sound decisions about bike positioning, help you solve issues around performance, injury, pain and discomfort, and help you get more out of cycling, without emptying your wallet at the same time.

Summary of methods of fit

- ▶ Traditional
- ▶ Observational
- ▶ Generic
- ▶ Individualised
  - ▪ Static
  - ▪ Dynamic

Traditional

Following CONI, the Italian cycling bible named after its publisher, and concentrating on riding position and foot placement, that is, with the ball of the foot on the spindle.

Advantages: quick and easy.
Disadvantages: does not take individual body type into account, forces the body to adapt to the bike.

Observational

Based on the beliefs of the individual about what a rider should look like.

Advantages: improves upon 'Traditional' by actually looking at the individual.
Disadvantages: no objective data, most riders end up looking the same.

Generic

Equation-based fit, using measurements of body segment lengths (CONI, Bioracer).

Advantages: improves on 'Observational' by measuring the body and recognising that proportions are important to bike fitting.
Disadvantages: static measurements, doesn't take into account the interaction between bike and rider.

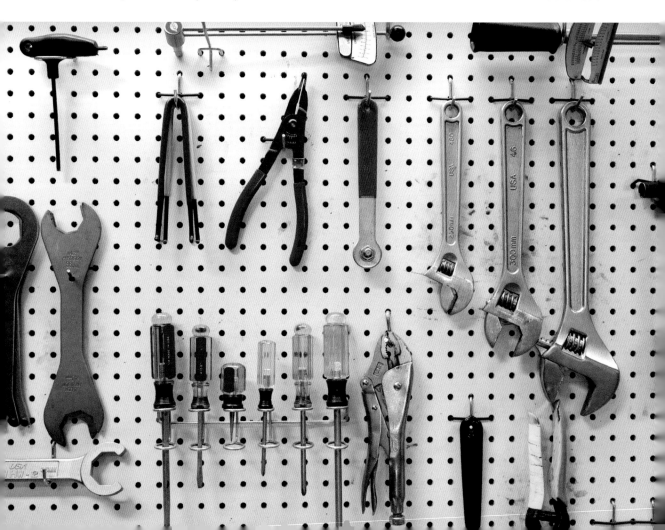

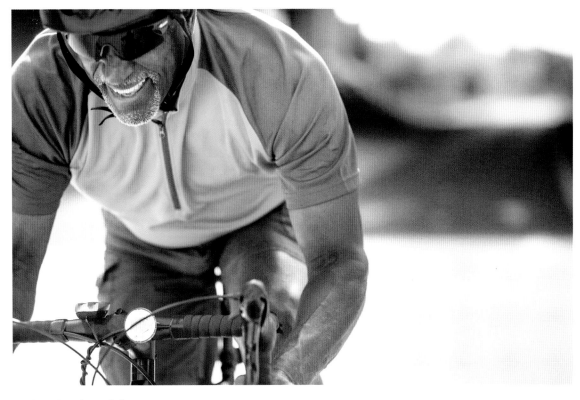

Individualised fit – static

Uses plumb bob (basically a piece of string with a weight at the end used to find vertical positions) and goniometry (a large protractor used to measure angles).

Advantages: uses joint angles to optimise fit.
Disadvantages: static nature can use only a theoretical riding position, not the true position(s) of the rider in motion.

Individualised fit – dynamic

Using either video or motion analysis data to adjust the bike to the rider while they are riding (in other words, while they are dynamic).

Advantages: uses objective data and the dynamic element provides a true reflection of someone riding.
Disadvantages: costly.

Neutral vs accommodative fitting

All of the above are tools to help you to bike fit. Of course, as with any tool, they can only be as good as the person using them. Just because someone has a £12,000 3D motion-capture system doesn't mean they will automatically do an optimal and appropriate bike fit for you. In fact, many in the know now consider the industry to be diverging into two categories: those who bike fit to a neutral set of ranges versus those who possess the skills and experience to complete an accommodative fit. Accommodative fitting is where one limitation of an individual is accommodated within the overall fit, perhaps at the slight expense of another parameter, but nevertheless giving a better overall fit, which remains safe.

I will use the term 'fit window' to mean the range of bike adjustments within which a rider will find suitable levels of comfort and performance. For the purposes of this book I describe the fit windows referenced to a neutral position for each of the different types of riding. I have alluded to lots of the common cases and reasons for fitting outside this window, but ultimately it may be beyond the scope of this book to help you complete a difficult fit accommodation. If you need an especially complicated fit, I recommend consulting an appropriately qualified practitioner.

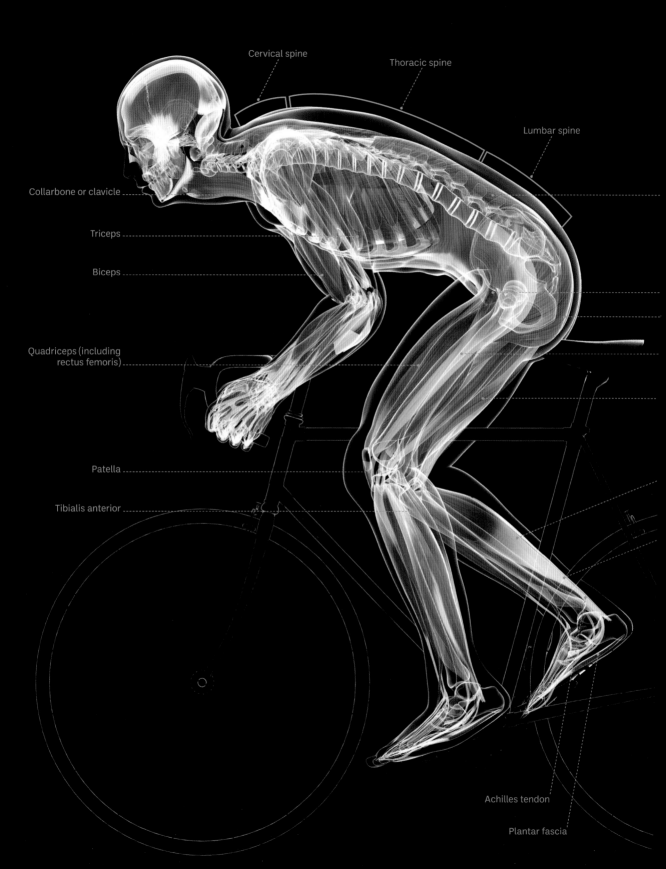

Cervical spine

Thoracic spine

Lumbar spine

Collarbone or clavicle

Triceps

Biceps

Quadriceps (including
rectus femoris)

Patella

Tibialis anterior

Achilles tendon

Plantar fascia

Long back muscles

Iliopsoas (hip flexor)

Gluteals

ITB (iliotibial band)

Hamstrings

Gastrocnemius

Soleus

02

Bike-related anatomy

Bike-related anatomy

In this chapter, we will examine the roles of certain muscles, joints and tendons in terms of cycling-force (torque) production, stability, posture, attenuation and ventilation. The overriding importance of power needs to be offset against your ability to hold and sustain a cycling posture or position. An understanding of which muscles are involved with both is very worthwhile.

Cycling is made possible by the coordination of a series of elements (muscles) that contract to create force, which is transferred through a series of levers (bones) via joints to create torque at the pedals. Muscles are essentially a vast array of sliding filaments. These filaments can hold static positions (isometrics), create force by shortening (concentric) or modify (attenuate) load by controlling the gain in muscle length (eccentrics).

Imagine holding a tin of beans in your right hand, with your elbow at a right angle to your body, while keeping absolutely still. The biceps muscle in your arm is not shortening or lengthening, but it is still working against gravity to hold the arm and tin of beans where it is. This is an isometric contraction. If you move the tin towards your shoulder by flexing your elbow, you shorten the biceps muscle. This is called a concentric contraction. If you then slowly lower your muscle in a controlled way (i.e. you lower your hand, rather than just letting it drop), your biceps is lengthening, but is still working to control the weight of the tin against gravity. This is an eccentric contraction.

Muscular actions and reactions are controlled by stimulation from nerves linked to the central nervous system (spinal cord and brain). Too often the neuro part of neuromuscular control is forgotten or overlooked. You can have a massive muscle, but if it is poorly controlled or coordinated it will not fulfil its potential. Our force-producing muscles are attached to our bones (or levers) by tendons, which are made up of fibrous material organised in a linear arrangement that is ideal for transferring force. All the muscles involved in cycling generate force in order to turn the pedal. 'Torque' is used to describe the force applied to a lever that results in rotation through an axis and is therefore appropriate for describing force in terms of pedalling.

Anatomy of the lower body

Joints have multiple axes of motion. The coordination of joints so that they move in the required way for a given task is a hugely complicated process involving many different elements, including muscles and nerves. Excessive (too lax) or limited (too stiff) motions can affect the joints above or below that motion in the kinetic chain. This is an important point to realise – that a movement in one part of the body affects the movement of the next like a series of levers.

For example, an observed irregular motion at the knee may be a result of irregularities in the foot or hip, and not necessarily isolated to the knee.

Hip

The hip is part of the pelvis and is the beginning of the torque chain for pedalling. The pelvis has a socket called the acetabulum that holds the head of the femur (or thigh-bone) to form the hip joint.

The skeletal system

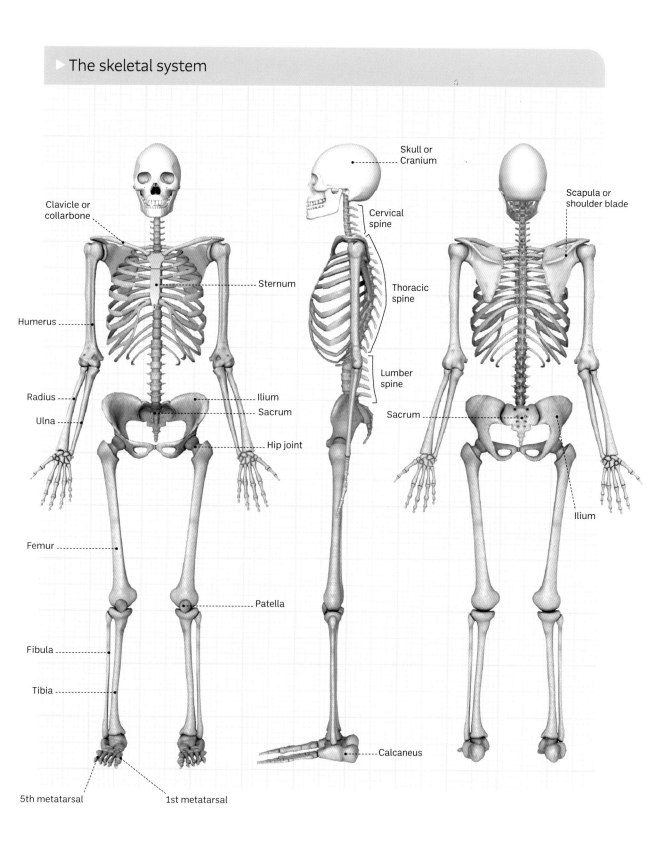

Skull or Cranium

Cervical spine

Thoracic spine

Lumber spine

Scapula or shoulder blade

Clavicle or collarbone

Sternum

Humerus

Radius

Ulna

Ilium

Sacrum

Hip joint

Sacrum

Ilium

Femur

Patella

Fibula

Tibia

Calcaneus

5th metatarsal

1st metatarsal

▶ The muscular system

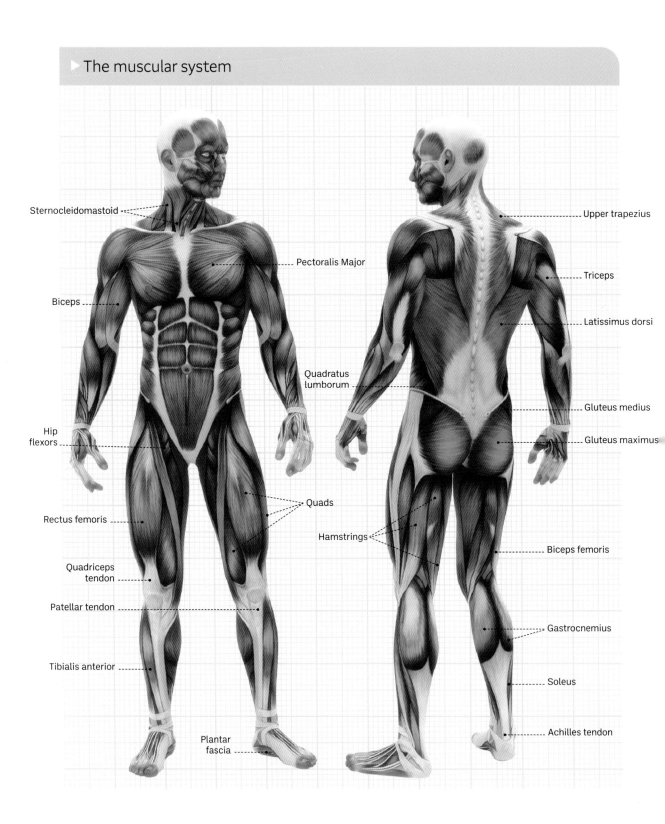

Sternocleidomastoid

Pectoralis Major

Biceps

Quadratus lumborum

Hip flexors

Quads

Rectus femoris

Quadriceps tendon

Patellar tendon

Tibialis anterior

Hamstrings

Plantar fascia

Upper trapezius

Triceps

Latissimus dorsi

Gluteus medius

Gluteus maximus

Biceps femoris

Gastrocnemius

Soleus

Achilles tendon

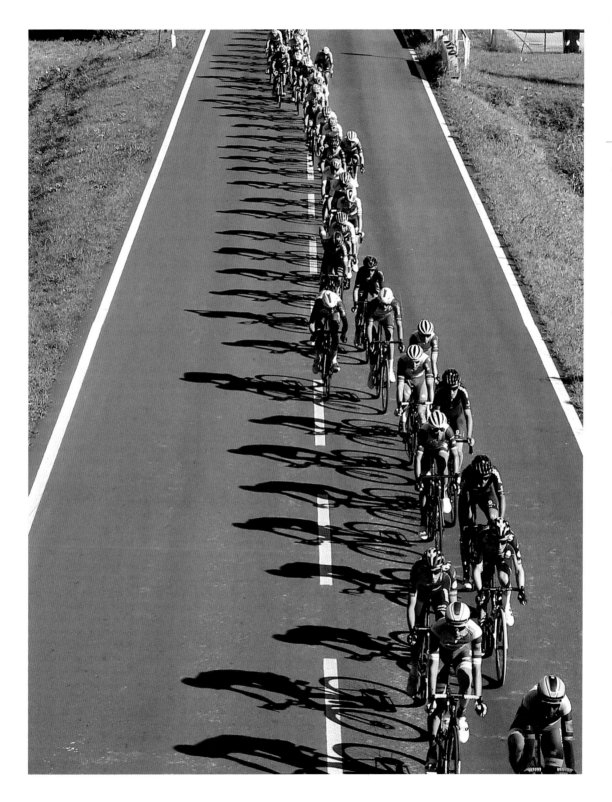

The hip joint allows and guides the motions of flexion, extension and rotation in the act of cycling. Irregularities in hip joint motion frequently limit the ability of the hip (and therefore the leg) to travel through the top part of the pedal stroke.

Due to its length, and the size and number of the muscles surrounding it (the gluteal, and quadriceps of the thigh/knee), large amounts of torque can be generated around the pelvis.

Pelvis

The pelvis is largely composed of two bony regions: the ischium and the ilium. These two bones articulate between the sacrum (the large triangular bone at the back of the pelvis) and the base of the spine at what is called the sacroiliac joint. Those who suffer from problems of the lower back may well have heard of this joint, as it is very close to the lumbar spine and can be the cause of pain. The ischium is an important part of the body in cycling because the hamstrings originate there, in the area known as the ischial tuberosity.

Also important for cycling is the group of muscles that make up the hip flexors and, in particular, the inner hip muscles known as the iliopsoas. These are made up of the iliacus, which fills the curve of the ilium on either side, and the two psoas muscles, which originate from the last three vertebrae. The hip flexors are an important muscle group in cycling, but their role is often misinterpreted and problems with them are frequently misdiagnosed. In fact, they contribute little (10–15 per cent) in the actual pulling up of the femur, except in maximal or sprint cycling, and become tight and/or painful, not due to their workload, but because of the very closed hip position cyclists sustain for long periods of time. See pages 115–17 for more on this.

Knee and upper leg

The knee consists of three bones: the femur (thigh), the tibia (shin) and the patella (kneecap). The femur projects downward to sit on top of the tibia and is the longest bone in the body. Torque is related to the size of the lever producing it: large forces through long levers, such as the femur, result in large torque. The patella acts as a fulcrum through which the force produced from the

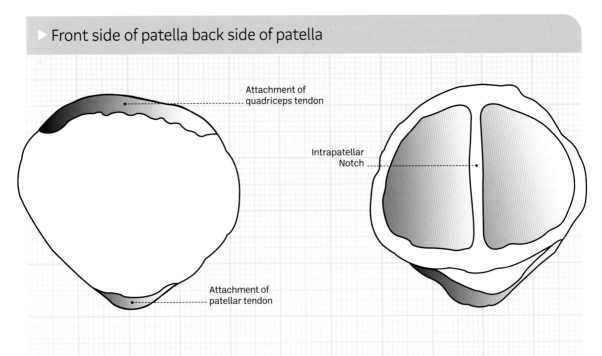

▶ Front side of patella back side of patella

Attachment of quadriceps tendon

Intrapatellar Notch

Attachment of patellar tendon

The patella (kneecap) has the job of working with the quadriceps tendon, in which it sits, to focus the transfer of force from the quads to the lower leg via the tibia. It moves smoothly across the base of the femur and knee joint.

quadriceps and glutei is transferred to the tibia, and ultimately to the pedal.

PATELLO-FEMORAL JOINT

The patello-femoral joint is the knee joint we most often talk about in cycling because of its role as the fulcrum, transferring push to the pedal. The picture below shows an oblique lateral view of the knee and the position of the patella on the femur. The patella is triangular in shape and is a 'sesamoid' bone – one that forms within a tendon. The bony prominence onto which the patellar tendon attaches is the tibial tuberosity.

The quadriceps tendon attaches the quadriceps to the patella and the patellar tendon attaches the patella to the tibia. The picture on page 28 shows the cartilage surface of the patella and the intra-patellar notch, which glides inside the groove created by the two condyles (or knuckles) of the end of the femur. The patello-femoral joint is a particularly smooth cartilage surface, with a coefficient of friction nine times that of ice sliding over ice. For this reason, a number of factors that can cause the patella to move too far out of the groove can cause pain.

The act of pedalling requires coordinated motions from many of the muscles of the lower body. Measuring the electrical activity within muscles (electromyography) during cycling confirms that the quadriceps and the glutei are the primary torque-producing muscles in pedalling. In other words, your thighs and your bum muscles are the key.

QUADRICEPS

The quadriceps is at the front of the thigh and is made up of four muscles: the vastus lateralis, the vastus medialis, the rectus femoris and the vastus intermedius (which sits under the rectus femoris). The quadriceps is an extender of the knee. When the quadriceps is engaged in a concentric (or shortening – remember the baked bean tin on page 24) manner, the knee straightens or extends. The rectus femoris is the only quadriceps muscle to cross the hip and knee, and is therefore termed a 'bi-articular' muscle, which can flex the hip. More often than not tightness in this muscle will be responsible for knee pain (in this case, patello-

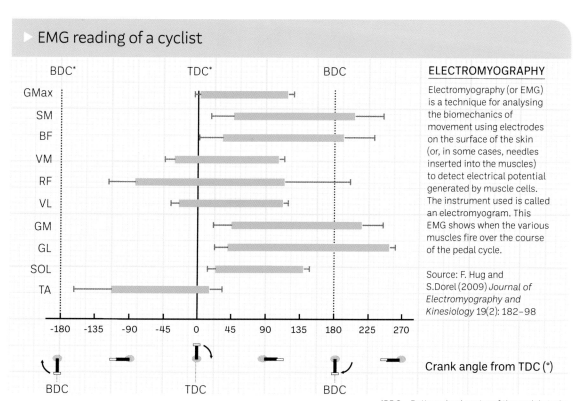

► EMG reading of a cyclist

ELECTROMYOGRAPHY

Electromyography (or EMG) is a technique for analysing the biomechanics of movement using electrodes on the surface of the skin (or, in some cases, needles inserted into the muscles) to detect electrical potential generated by muscle cells. The instrument used is called an electromyogram. This EMG shows when the various muscles fire over the course of the pedal cycle.

Source: F. Hug and S. Dorel (2009) *Journal of Electromyography and Kinesiology* 19(2): 182–98

Crank angle from TDC (°)

*BDC = Bottom dead centre of the pedal stroke
TDC = top dead centre of the pedal stroke

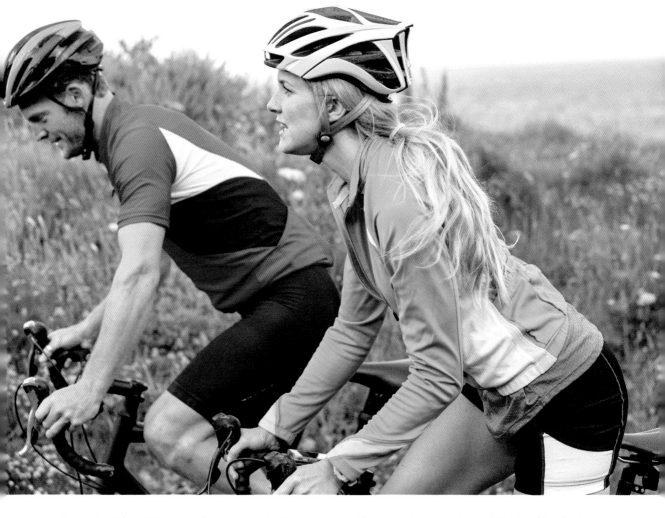

femoral pain), as it increases the compressive force around the joint when it is too short or not functioning as well as it should. The extension or propulsive force couple is completed by the gluteus maximus or hip extender.

HAMSTRINGS

The hamstrings, comprised of the biceps femoris, semimembranosis and the semitendinosis, stabilise the knee during the bottom of the pedal stroke and help direct the leg through the back part of the pedal stroke.

Lower leg

In cycling, the lower leg is responsible for transferring force from the quadriceps and glutei to the pedal. It consists of the tibia, fibula, ankle and foot. The ankle is made up of the talus, which sits on top of the calcaneus (heel bone). The foot is generally separated into three different regions: rear foot, midfoot and forefoot. Irregular motion from the foot can originate from any of these three regions. The long bones of the foot are known as metatarsals and it is important to know where they are as they are used to position the foot correctly on the pedal.

EMG studies show that, while calf muscles do not add significantly to power created further up the kinetic chain, they do work hard to help the lower leg stay in position and better transfer power to the pedal. If they are not working effectively power can be lost, so they shouldn't be dismissed as irrelevant just because their net contribution might seem less than their size suggests.

Two muscles help to stabilise the foot so that it can create a rigid lever to move the pedal – the gastrocnemius and the soleus. These muscles collectively form the calf muscle. The gastrocnemius has two heads, originating above the knee on the femur and running down to the calcaneus. It combines with the soleus to make the Achilles tendon, which is common to both muscles. The soleus is deep to (further from the skin than) the gastrocnemius and helps make the foot a rigid lever to the pedal. It originates just below the knee (on the tibia and fibula) and travels down to the calcaneus through the Achilles tendon.

Other muscles that support the foot include the ankle invertors, evertors and dorsiflexors. These muscles of the foot and ankle originate on the lower leg and support the arches of the foot.

Anatomy of the trunk and back

While the legs do most of the work, they still need a strong base of support, which is where the trunk and back muscles come in. Studies of the back muscles of endurance cyclists show increased activity in the back muscles when the load to the pedals increases.

Muscles of the back are arranged in a series. In the lower back are deep, small muscles called the multifidi and a larger muscle called the quadratus lumborum. These muscles help stabilise the spine under lateral and rotational loads.

The next layer of muscles of the back are the longissimus. These muscles are extensors over multiple segments of the back and help maintain posture and stability while cycling.

Abdominal musculature is mostly used to keep the trunk stable in brief moments under high force. If you are cycling under aerobic conditions you will usually use your abdominal muscles for diaphragmatic breathing.

Originating from the upper back and shoulder are the trapezius and the latissimus dorsi. These are important as stabilisers in cycling because they fix the arms, allowing them to work as anchors. As you push the left pedal, your right arm fixes and pulls on the handlebar,

through the action of the right latissimus dorsus, to stabilise you, and vice versa. Think about when you are pushing hard, climbing or sprinting: you can really feel your arms working in this way. It still happens at gentler paces, but is not as noticeable.

The biceps also acts as a stabilising muscle in conjunction with the latissimus dorsi, again counteracting torque production from the legs, stabilising the torso by pulling into the handlebar. The right arm counterbalances the torso from torque produced from the left leg, and vice versa.

Attenuation

Attenuation is essentially load absorption: think of the action of a shock absorber. The main muscles soaking up impact from the road surface while cycling are the triceps and calf muscles. Eccentric muscle action allows loads to be smoothed out or 'attenuated'. Load attenuation of the triceps from handlebar vibration and loading protects the neck and shoulder. Load attenuation from the calf muscles allows the torso and hip/knee to stay stable over bumpy surfaces as well.

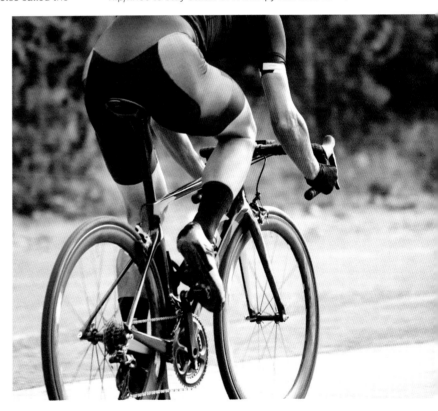

Posture

Posture is the maintenance of a certain body position and requires appropriate joint mobility, joint/muscle coordination and muscular endurance. Limits in any of these elements can result in postural irregularities. Good posture on the bicycle requires good flexibility through the hamstrings and the glutei muscles: this allows the pelvis to roll forward, keeping the back in a straight position while reaching for the handlebars.

One major factor limiting the back's ability to remain relatively straight while on a bicycle is thoracic immobility: lack of movement in the middle of the spine normally results in the spine flexing too much. Excessive spinal flexion while on a bicycle will limit breathing and compromise your ability to stabilise your spine for torque production to the pedals.

Ventilation

Ventilation is simply the act of getting air into and out of the lungs. It is crucial for the endurance athlete that this process is as efficient as possible. The lungs reside within a bony cage created by the ribs, which are anchored in the body through a tight articulation to the thoracic spine. There are anatomical and bicycle limiters to ventilation. An example of an anatomical limiter to ventilation would be being too flexed through the thoracic spine (that is, bent forward), not allowing the ribcage to expand sufficiently. Examples of bicycle position limiters may be compact aero positions that compromise breathing, or rearward saddle tilts that require spinal bending to maintain a seated position on the saddle.

Ventilation for the endurance athlete is most effectively performed through diaphragmatic breathing, in which contraction and relaxation of the diaphragm pulls and pushes air from the lungs. Secondary muscles of ventilation include the intercostals (between the ribs), the abdominal musculature, the trapezius, the levator scapulae and the scalenes. If diaphragmatic breathing is compromised these secondary muscles can become chronically overworked leading to myofascial type pain (i.e. pain between the muscle and the muscle covering). This is often seen in the upper neck and shoulder muscles.

▶ Nerves of the foot

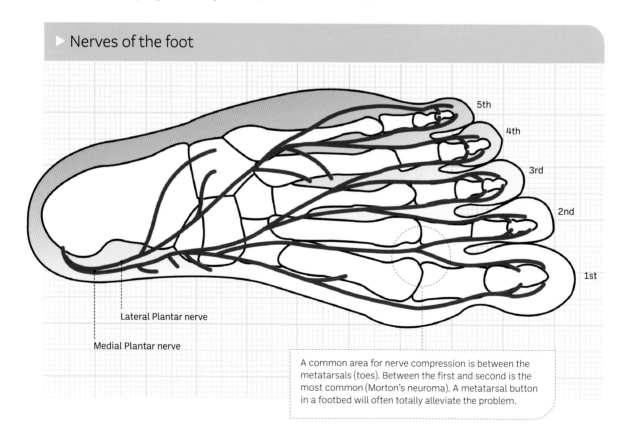

5th
4th
3rd
2nd
1st

Lateral Plantar nerve

Medial Plantar nerve

A common area for nerve compression is between the metatarsals (toes). Between the first and second is the most common (Morton's neuroma). A metatarsal button in a footbed will often totally alleviate the problem.

Contact points

Simply put, these are the points at which your body touches the bike. We will look at them in more detail later, but it's helpful to examine the anatomical reasons why they are so important to get set correctly.

The three primary anatomical contact points to the bicycle can be sources of numbness and pain. These are: foot to pedal, hand to handlebar and pelvis to saddle. Numbness, weakness and pain can arise when vascular (blood vessel) and neural (nerve) tissues have irregular loading, resulting in compression.

Foot to pedal

This view of the bottom of the foot shown here exhibits neural distribution. Poor cleat position or irregular support or compression of the foot can result in tissue damage. Amid a complex vascular system of veins, which pump blood towards the heart, and arterioles, which carry oxygenated blood from the lungs to the muscles, are the nerves, depicted in red in the diagram. Note their trajectory between the metatarsal heads.

Nerves are a primary site of bicycle-related foot pain.

Hand to handlebar

The two main nerves that supply the hand are the median nerve and the ulnar nerve. These nerves pass through two tunnels as they enter the hand region: the carpal tunnel (median) and the tunnel of Guyon (ulnar). Irregular positioning of the hand to the handlebar can include being positioned too widely, leading to the fingers splaying, or too much weight being placed on the hand due to the overall position. Such positioning can compress nerves, resulting in pain, numbness and weakness in certain muscles. Compression of the median nerve will result in numbness of the first three fingers and half of the fourth, while the ulnar nerve will affect the lateral half of the fourth finger and all of the fifth.

Pelvis to saddle

The saddle region as related to the pelvis has pressure-sensitive arteries and nerves. Irregular compressive loading for anatomical or bike fit reasons will result in numbness, pain and loss of tissue function.

▶ Nerves of the hand

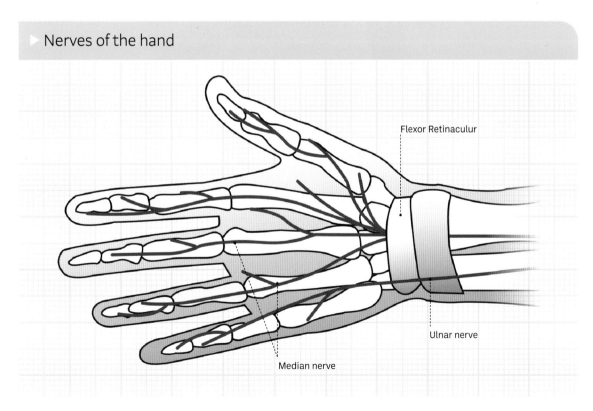

Flexor Retinaculur

Ulnar nerve

Median nerve

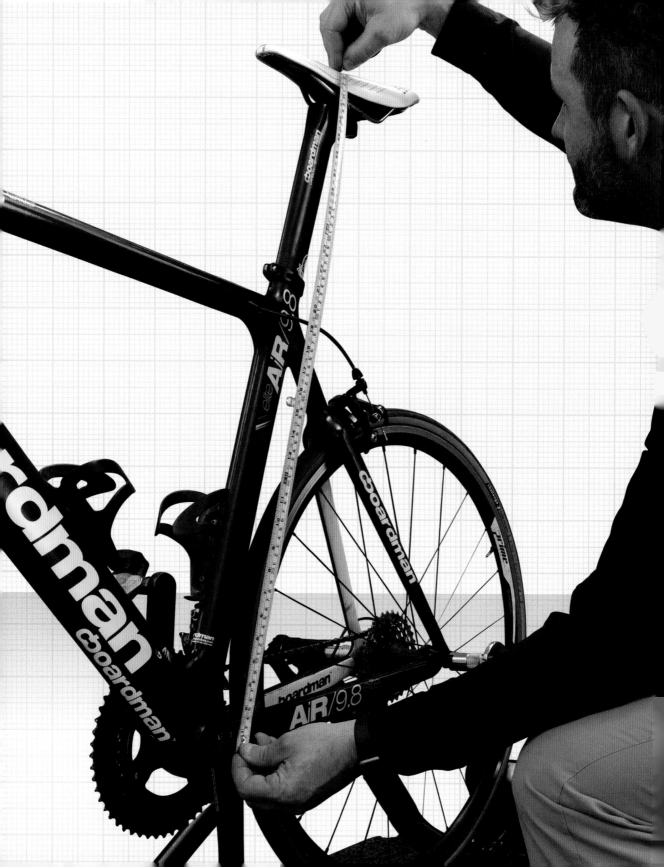

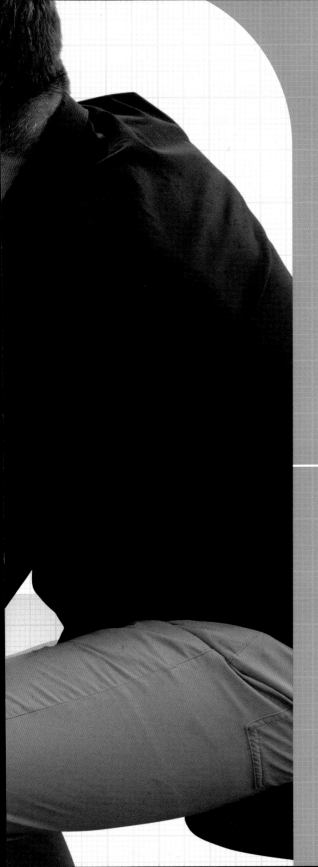

03

The bike fit window

The bike fit window

People often ask me what the perfect position is. My response is: for what? The perfect position varies depending on what you are looking for: power, comfort or sustainability, or aerodynamics.

You could easily justify setting a bike position separately for each, but in fact all positions are a compromise between these four criteria. The position is skewed towards what the rider wants, but restricted by what they can handle. So what's the perfect compromise position? I don't think it exists for longer than a day – at the most – and it is therefore irrelevant. On any given day somebody's perfect bike position will be different to the day before. Take one key parameter: a person's ability to touch his or her toes is a combination of their various 'segmental flexibilities' – at the knee, hips (hamstrings) and lumbo-pelvic region. With age and injury we all trend towards becoming less flexible and stiffer, but we do so at differing rates. Over 50 per cent of us suffer from some form of lower back pain and this is often associated with stiffness – and our sedentary lifestyles are partly responsible.

I could fit you to your perfect position at 8am on

▶ Parts of a standard bike

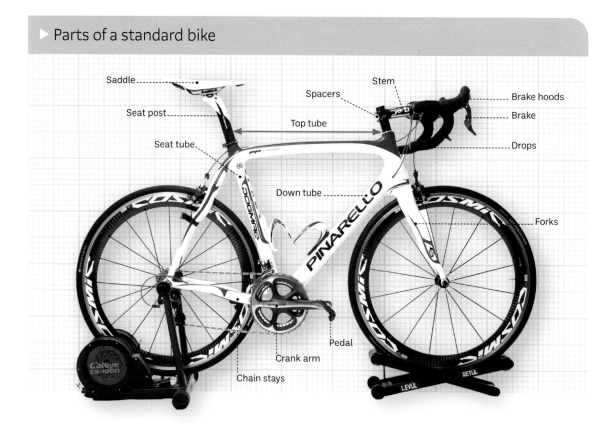

Saddle

Stem

Spacers

Brake hoods

Seat post

Top tube

Brake

Seat tube

Drops

Down tube

Forks

Pedal

Crank arm

Chain stays

a Friday morning after you had spent a long week at work sitting at an office desk. The position would take account of your relative inflexibility in the lower back and to accommodate this it would be more conservative, more upright and with the handlebars up. But if you came in after a weekend free of work and full of riding, your ideal position would have changed: the lumbar spine might well be more flexible relative to Friday morning and your 'perfect position' would have to reflect this: it would be more aggressive, less upright, with the handlebars lower. Even the quality of a night's sleep can be enough to change someone's 'perfect' position.

The same is true of professional riders coming off long mountain stages, suffering after sustained climbing slung back in the saddle for hours upon hours. Their ideal position changes when they enter the flat stages of a race like the Tour de France and many are attentive enough to have different bike set-ups accordingly.

For this reason, I prefer to think of the 'bike fit window' instead of a perfect position and I aim to fit

to this. I believe the phrase was first coined and made popular by Andy Pruitt, but it describes perfectly how we should envisage our fluid relationship with the bike. Imagine your three major measurements and contact points with the bike: saddle height, handlebars and foot/cleat. The fit window is between the maximum and minimum for each variable. For example, I normally describe people's saddle height (assuming it is roughly correct) as high or low within the fit window. Their lowest acceptable saddle height might be 78cm, and the top 79.5cm. Beyond these boundaries the height becomes less than ideal, but within this zone someone can be perfectly comfortable and perform. Your saddle height on a Friday after work would be at the bottom of your zone (reflecting your relative inflexibility at that time), but by Monday it would be at the top – your fit window changes due to an improvement in flexibility.

The fit window is more than just that, however. It's the relationship between these key foot-to-pedal contact points. You'll often hear saddle height and foot-to-pedal described as the positional height of a rider, while the handlebars give the positional length because

▶ The balance between height and length of posture

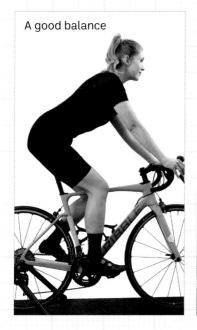

A good balance

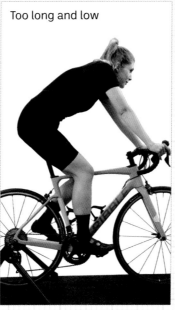

Too long and low

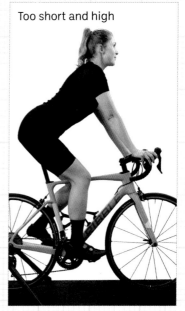

Too short and high

their location determines how far you reach: lower handlebars mean you have to lean further forward. The fore/aft position of the saddle affects length as well and we will discuss this later (see pages 48–50). Most fitting concentrates on getting the back-end height optimal first, as this is where power is derived – the engine room, so to speak. What I like to call the cockpit – the front end – is then set up making sure the rider is balanced, the back angle is comfortable and the arms are able to relax at the elbows. All this determines whether the head position is comfortable – whether the rider can comfortably look up the road extending from the neck.

The balance of bike fitting from the side-on view at first principles is simply this – getting the height of the engine room and position of the cockpit so the tilt of the rider is optimal. Get this wrong and the rider is either tilted too far forward or too far backwards.

Bottom and top dead centre

The terms 'bottom dead centre' (BDC) and 'top dead centre' (TDC) are a nice technical shorthand for the position of the leg at the very bottom and the very top, respectively, of the pedal motion. If one leg is at BDC, the other leg will be at TDC, and the pedals will sit directly over and under the centre of the crankset, and the crank arms will be vertical.

Joint angles

The bike fit window can be expressed in terms of the physical measurement of key distances over the bike, such as saddle height and reach to handlebars. The parameters that determine those measurements are the rider's interaction with the bike. These are best expressed as the joint angles the rider adopts to ride the bike in a particular position. By joint angle I simply mean the angle of the bend of, say, the knee – for

▶ Retŭl basic measurement averages and ranges for a road bike

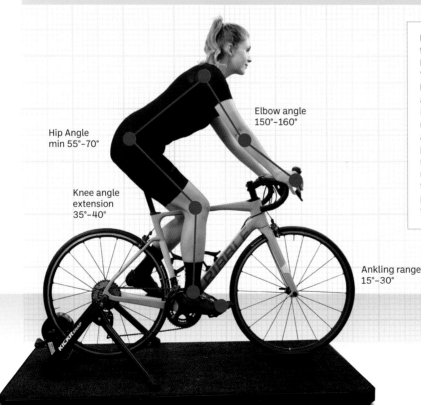

In this book the ranges quoted for joint angles refer to the Retül standard joint ranges. You can discover more about how these ranges are calculated at www.retul.com. Note that in the diagram 'ankling range' refers to the amount the ankle angle should vary during the pedal cycle, and that 'hip angle min.' refers to this angle at its most acute, for instance for the left leg here. Compare with page 143 for time trial and triathlon bikes.

Elbow angle
150°–160°

Hip Angle
min 55°–70°

Knee angle
extension
35°–40°

Ankling range
15°–30°

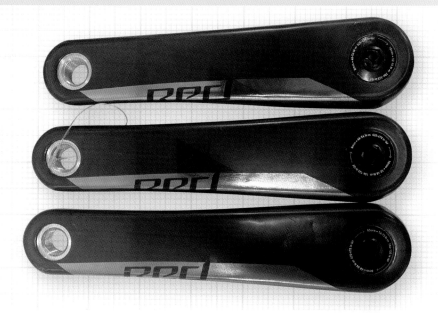

example a knee extension at bottom dead centre (BDC) of a pedal stroke of 35 degrees. Many keen riders know that there are optimal ranges for these joint angles, outside which the fit becomes less than ideal (i.e. injurious, uncomfortable and performance-limiting). I use joint angles, not formulae, to optimise bike fit. The diagram shows the fit window for a road bike from a joint angle perspective.

How to get into your bike fit window

If you're coming to me for a bike fit, chances are you've already spent a fair amount of time riding, but you'd be surprised what I see in terms of position, even with the best riders. When I first analyse a new cyclist, I take them through a process that has dynamic fit at its heart. Static fit is fine up to a point, but dynamic fit – where you can measure someone's knee position relative to their foot while they are actually cycling – is the gold standard. The goals and the essential rules of the fit window are the same, but this is a different (and I believe better) way of getting there.

Crank length

I've had a suspicion that crank length is the elephant in the bike fit studio for a long time and, although we saw the aero benefits of shortening cranks for time trials and pursuit during my time with British Cycling, since working with a wide range of riders I've really seen the impact it can have on both comfort and power production. This almost Damascene realisation that I've come to regarding crank length is probably the most significant and impactful thing I've learned since working with a broader range of cyclists, and it's why this subject has gone from a short side note to being front and centre in this edition.

I would say that cranks are the most common component I change for riders who come to me for a fit and the impact is often a game changer. If you think about a bike, the only point that relates to position that doesn't move is the bottom bracket. In fact, not wishing to simplify my job, but bike fit is all about rotating riders around the bottom bracket. A time triallist will be rotated right forward, a road rider back a bit and a mountain biker even further back, and bike fit is just about achieving and accommodating this rotation.

In the middle of this are the cranks, so it's only logical that they're going to have an effect.

The leverage myth

There's a long-held belief in cycling that for increased leverage and torque you need longer cranks, and in disciplines such as pursuit you'll still see riders fitting 175mm+ cranks because of this. Even coaches at the highest level still cling to this fallacy that longer cranks equals more power.

In the last decade, though, a number of studies have shown that increased crank length has little if any impact on power production. One such study found that, for sub-maximal cycling, you'd have to go as low as 80mm and as high as 320mm to have a significant effect on power production. In this case, sub-maximal basically referred to any cycling that wasn't the opening two pedal strokes out of the gate on a team sprint.

So if changing crank length has no impact on power production, but it can improve comfort, aerodynamics and other areas, why wouldn't you look to change it? Why would you want to pedal a large circle rather than a smaller one? The analogy I often use with clients is, if you had a 1m plyometric box and a 15cm step and I offered you £100 to jump onto one a hundred times, which would you pick? Of course you'd want to pedal a smaller circle and shift any problems to your gears rather than your ankles, knees, hips and lower back.

Are you a candidate for shorter cranks?

I'll put my head on the bike fit block here and say that, regardless of height, almost all cyclists would benefit from shorter cranks. The bike industry really needs to wake up to this and 165mm really needs to become the standard. There are a number of pointers, though, that indicate shorter cranks could help you.

If you struggle to maintain higher cadences no matter how low your gearing, simply dropping from 175mm to 165mm will increase your cadence. Track riders tend to ride 165mm cranks due to clearance round the steep banking, but, because of these shorter cranks, are able to sustain higher cadences.

If you have a history of knee pain or injury, shorter cranks will mean reduced knee flexion to get over the top of the pedal stroke and therefore less strain on the joint.

Very few humans are symmetrical and this often manifests in cyclists as pain or discomfort on one side. This could be, for example, right side saddle pain combined with left side knee pain. The longer the crank, the more any asymmetry is going to be amplified and, conversely, if you shorten the crank, the less the impact will be.

If you tend to suffer from back pain on the bike this is often related to a tightening of the hip flexors. If you shorten your cranks, this will open up your hips, your knees won't have to come as high and this will help to relax your back.

If you bounce on the saddle, especially at higher cadences, this can be an indicator that your body is struggling to accommodate too-long cranks. Similarly, do you suffer from saddle soreness despite trying all of the usual steps (see page 119) to remedy it? With shorter cranks, peaks in saddle pressure are reduced and I've seen many riders experience a significant reduction in saddle discomfort by reducing crank length.

Does your bike feel too long and that you're reaching for the bars despite the sizing seeming to be correct?

Do you need to spin to win?

Popularised by Lance Armstrong – who we now know had some other 'helpers' as well – and more recently Chris Froome, pedalling on the road at cadences above 100rpm became widely touted as the most efficient way to pedal. If only it was this simple. It may well have been for Lance and Chris, but to suggest this works for everyone is to ignore the many components that make up pedalling efficiency. For example, cadence is affected by crank length and gear selection. Research shows that the optimal cadence metabolically (in terms of energy expended for work done) is 60rpm, yet studies show that most people's preferred cadence is around 90rpm. This is probably a trade-off between metabolic efficiency and force production, and where the balance of those two lies is different for different individuals. Interestingly, as power increases so does your optimal cadence for holding it. Elite cyclists can hold 100rpm relatively easily, because they are well trained.

This could be because you're sitting higher and further back in order to be able to accommodate too-long cranks. Moving forward will solve the reach issue, but, because of the crank length, you'll feel cramped in your hips.

I could go on, but the bottom line is that I'm yet to meet a rider who wouldn't benefit from shorter cranks. They just give you more freedom within the fit window and, whether your priority is getting lower and going faster or simply being able to ride longer and stay comfortable, shorter cranks could well be the solution.

Are oval chainrings better than circular ones?

It is currently hard to say either way on this issue, but oval chainrings aren't a particularly new concept, with Shimano touting their BioPace chainrings in the 1990s, although they had them misaligned by 90 degrees!

In some ways an oval chainring makes sense, because it decreases the dead-zone area of the pedal stroke where you are not creating positive power. Others argue there's no such thing as a free lunch and that the benefit of extending your leg for longer, which is in effect what a oval chainring does, is offset by the longer return in flexion experienced. Despite lots of research, to date no gains have ever been demonstrated in a scientific study. It may be that different shapes suit different riders. We just do not know currently. What is interesting to note is that despite being used by a number of top level pros for a number of years, including Chris Froome, watching the first time trial stage of the 2021 Tour de France, I didn't see a single one.

Going shorter?

Unfortunately, the bike industry is still catching up with the science and probably has a load of 175mm cranks that they still have to get rid of! This means, for a while

yet, if you're buying an off-the-peg bike, chances are the cranks will be too long.

Fortunately, a number of bike brands now allow you to spec different components and this is also a big

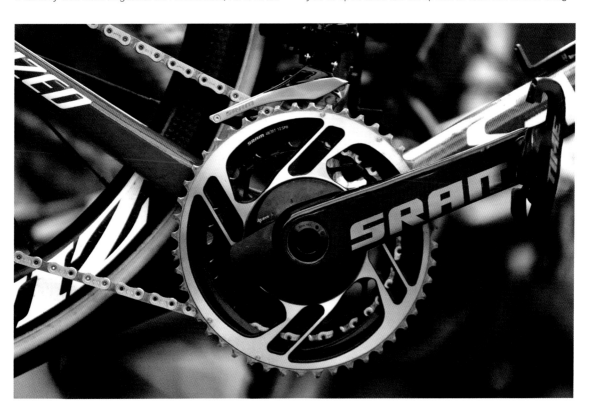

advantage of building a bike frame up, especially if you know you have specific fit requirements. The big three groupset manufacturers – Shimano, Campagnolo and SRAM – all offer 165mm cranks, but they can take a bit of finding. A number of manufacturers go down to 150mm and I've found Rotor to be one of the easiest to source. There are very few riders who'd need to go shorter than this, but I've done a bike fit for an acromegalic cyclist who was struggling with 150mm cranks and we had to go down the custom-built route.

Now I can understand that, if you've got a fleet of bikes with expensive groupsets and maybe even crank- or spider-based power meters, a wholesale change of cranks is going to be an expensive business. If you haven't got any issues, then maybe just experiment over time as and when you replace groupsets. However, if you are struggling with your position, injury or discomfort and just can't seem to solve the problem, it could be as simple as changing your cranks.

Saddle

Seat height is the Holy Grail for power. It's often argued that it is the most important cycle position setting and I have to agree – many other positioning recommendations, say of the handlebars or pedals, are actually trying to correct a suboptimal seat height.

> Relative seat height can be altered in many different ways other than merely moving the saddle up or down. Any change to the bike set-up that changes the distance from the seat to the pedal effectively changes seat height.

Optimum saddle height is described by the natural position of the leg fully extended at the BDC of the pedal stroke. This in turn depends on angles of the knee and ankle. A knee extension angle of 35-40 degrees is optimal for the average rider. Professional cyclists can be seen using angles of up to 30 degrees.

As with all positioning we have to create a

▶ Knee angles

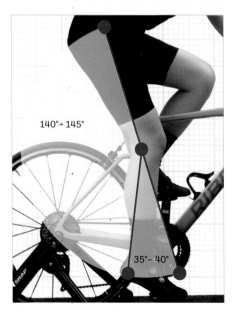

A knee extension angle of 140–145 degrees (which in the trade we refer to as 35–40 degrees, being the angle of deviation from a straight leg) is optimal for the average rider.

▶ Power vs saddle height

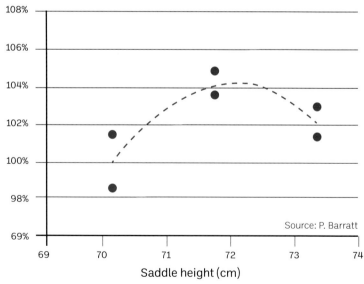

Source: P. Barratt

As saddle height increases so does power until a point where it drops again. Just before this drop is the optimal saddle height for power production. It is less likely to be optimal for comfort.

compromise between the variables of power, comfort and injury avoidance. The graph here clearly demonstrates what we know well: that there is an optimum saddle height for power production.

If the saddle is too low, the quadriceps and glutei cannot generate enough power as they never reach their optimal length. Too high and the knee is overreaching, too extended and the leg loses its grip on the pedal therefore producing less power.

The optimal saddle height for power has to be a goal that you work towards. These saddle heights are often at the very top end of the fit window I mentioned earlier and require knee extension angles at BDC of 30-25 degrees.

The main limiting factor for most of us in achieving this angle is our hamstring flexibility. Tight hamstrings inhibit knee extension and prevent us from rolling our pelvis forward, so a lot of us will never achieve beyond 40-degree knee extension at BDC.

Placing someone in their optimal seat height for power alone without reference to their flexibility means that they will feel strain and pain at the back of the

knee, and may, over time, develop an overuse injury.

Too low a saddle height, on the other hand, increases the compressive forces on the knee cap, as the leg comes over top dead centre (TDC) and pushes down. This can also cause pain and injury.

So if you want to ride safely and comfortably saddle height needs to be a compromise, accommodating all of these parameters. Ideally you should aim to get in the middle of the fit window.

Saddle height – static methods

One of the simplest ways to establish your saddle height statically is the heel to pedal at BDC method, advocated by many over the years. When you are starting out in cycling this is a simple method to get you in the right ballpark for saddle height.

Simply sit on your bike, on your rollers or turbo trainer if you have them (or just lean against a wall), and pedal backwards with your heel on the centre of the pedal. If your saddle height is correct your knee should be completely straight as you reach BDC

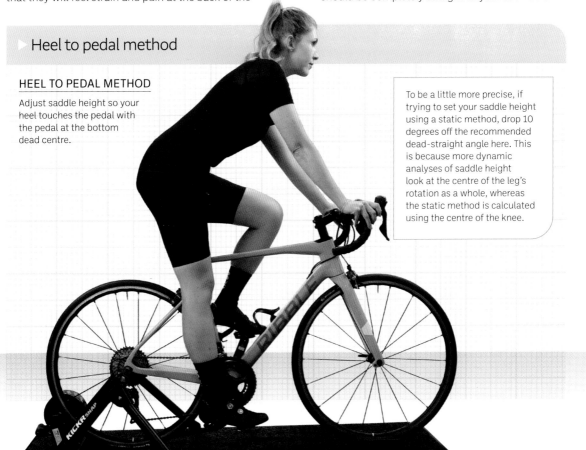

▶ Heel to pedal method

HEEL TO PEDAL METHOD
Adjust saddle height so your heel touches the pedal with the pedal at the bottom dead centre.

To be a little more precise, if trying to set your saddle height using a static method, drop 10 degrees off the recommended dead-straight angle here. This is because more dynamic analyses of saddle height look at the centre of the leg's rotation as a whole, whereas the static method is calculated using the centre of the knee.

(the 6 o'clock position). If it is still bent or your heel completely loses contact with the pedal, adjust your saddle height accordingly.

The drawback to the static method is that there are a few factors it doesn't take account of, for example the thickness of your cycling shoes, the position of the cleats on the shoes, how far backwards your saddle is set and your pedalling style.

Pedalling style

I said earlier that saddle height is defined by the 'nature of the leg at full extension'. This consists of not just the

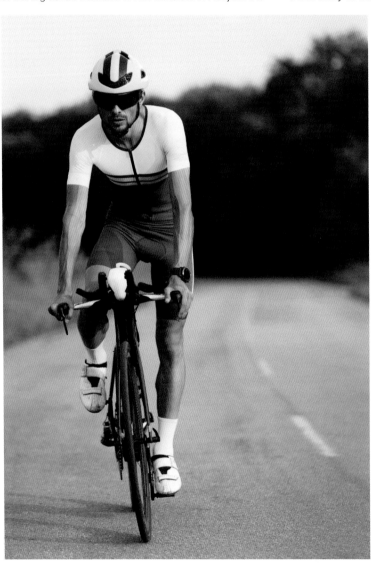

knee angle, but also the angle of the ankle. Pedalling styles differ massively across the cycling population; someone who pedals with their toe pointed right down can achieve a higher saddle height without altering their knee angle, compared to someone who pedals heel down. At the extremes of pedalling style you can't fit solely according to knee angle.

Formulae

I mentioned these briefly in my introduction. Many 'magic bullet' formulae exist, but the one you're most likely to know about was popularised by Greg LeMond and his coach in the early 1980s. You measure your inseam: stand with your back against a wall, place a flat object similar to a saddle under your groin and recreate the pressure exerted on your saddle while riding. Measure the distance between the floor and your crotch in centimetres. Multiply this figure by 0.883 and you have your saddle height, defined as the distance measured between the bottom bracket of the bike to the top of the saddle in line with the seat tube. This method has got many riders into the fit window for their saddle height.

The drawback of formulae is that they pay no respect to the nuances of the individual: flexibility, pedalling style or genetics (they will not help someone with long limbs and a short torso, or vice versa). Therefore, this method cannot help everyone to establish an optimal saddle height.

Goniometry

Another way to set your saddle height is to use a long-armed goniometer to measure your knee angle. Put the leg in the BDC (or 6 o'clock pedal position). Then measure between three key points:

the greater trochanter at the hip (the widest bony mass on the side of your hip), the centre of rotation at the knee and the bony mass on the outside of the ankle joint. The knee angle that will enable most people to ride in comfort without injury while still producing power is ideally 25-35 degrees.

The main drawback is that this is a static measurement requiring little attention to detail to perform and it may fail to take account of the actual riding or foot position. This can lead to a suboptimal setting once you actually start to ride.

Saddle height – dynamic methods

To date, by far the best method of setting saddle height is dynamic measure. In other words, recording the positions of someone's knee and ankle angle while they are actually riding. A system such as Retül can take thousands of data point measurements over a short time and average out the angles. In the hands

of a skilled bike fitter this data can be combined with an appreciation of the rider's body limitations to place someone bang in the middle of their specific fit window.

Saddle setback or fore/aft

Once you have established your saddle height, it's important to get the setback or fore/aft position of the saddle right. This parameter is key in optimising pedal power, preventing injury and setting the overall balance of the rider on the bike.

Saddle setback determines the position of your knee and hips in relation to the foot-to-pedal interface. If the knees and hip are too far behind the foot/pedal in the 3 o'clock position, it is harder to generate optimal power when pedalling.

Conversely if they are too far forward, with the knee in front of the foot/pedal interface in the 3 o'clock crank position, there is an increased risk of developing knee problems due to the increased forces placed on the kneecap.

▶ Lemond method

INSEAM FORMULA

Multiply the inseam height by 0.883 for saddle height, according to this method. It can work for some, but not everyone has the same body proportions.

▶ Goniometer

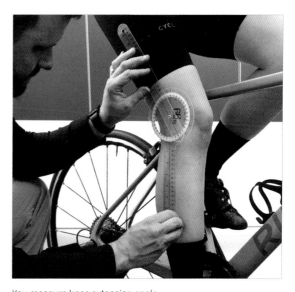

You measure knee extension angle on the bike to set your saddle height.

Source: bikefit.com ©BikeFit LLC

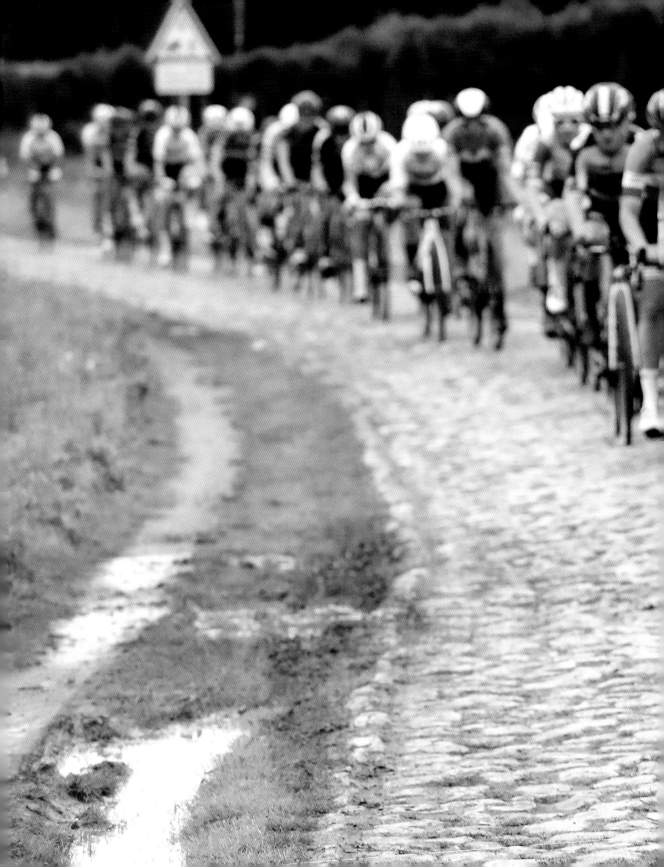

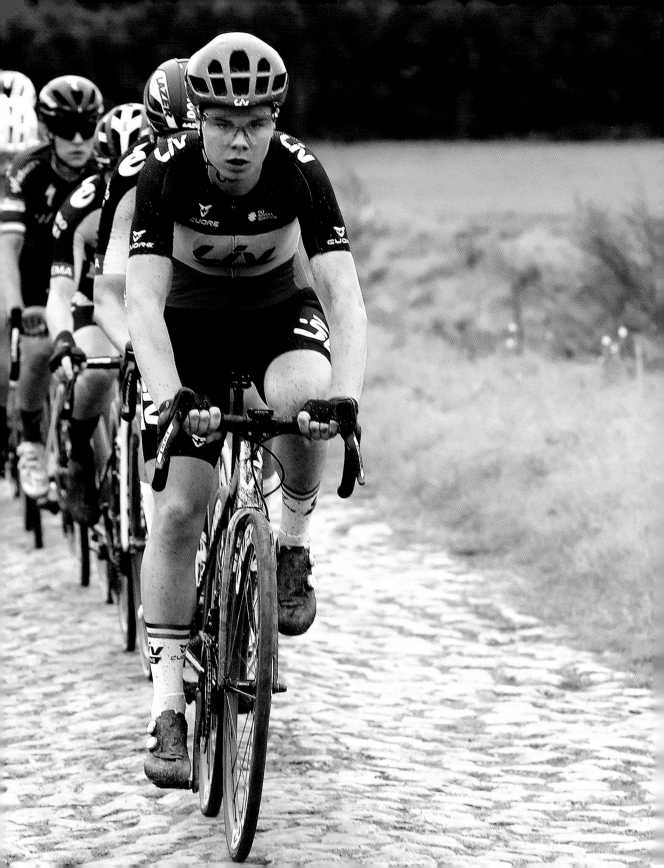

Try for yourself. Sit almost off the back of your saddle and try pedalling – it's hard because the point you are trying to push and control is further away. Now sit right forward, with only the very back of your bottom touching the saddle. This feels uncomfortable and bunched up, with the kneecaps under too much strain. In the fit window your saddle setback allows you to generate force from the quads and glutes, and to feel in control and free from risk of overuse injury.

Getting this coordinate of bike fit right also has a significant role in setting the correct balance of the rider on the bike. Overall balance is a sum of the relationship between all the fit points, of which this is one. If the saddle setback is too large, you will have the majority of your weight towards the back end of the bike, making handling lighter and less controlled at the front. This can be dangerous, for example when descending at speed through corners. If you are sitting too far back, you may have a very large distance to reach the handlebars unless you have taken care to adjust the handlebars appropriately. This can lead to pain and injury from overstretched tissues. If the saddle is too far forward, the rider can experience too much weight on the hands and wrists and develop issues, the classic being ulnar neuropathy (see page 135)

How to set saddle setback – static

The 'KOPS' method stands for Knee Over Pedal Spindle. And that's exactly what it does – establish the correct setback position by attempting to place the knee directly above the pedal spindle with the cranks at the 3 o'clock position.

Traditionally, a plumb line is dropped down from the tibial tuberosity (the bottom of the knee), and the saddle is adjusted until the line bisects the pedal spindle. There are a number of problems, conceptual and practical, with this method, well documented by other authors (for instance, see the article online by Keith Bontrager called

▶ Knee too far in front of the pedal

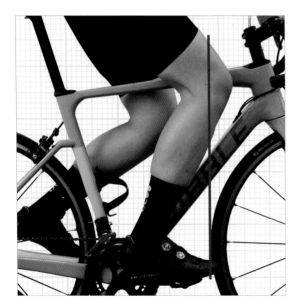

Note the postion of the front of the knee in relation to the foot. In this 'knee forward of foot' position there is an increase in the forces compressing the patella.

▶ KOPS: Knee Over Pedal Spindle

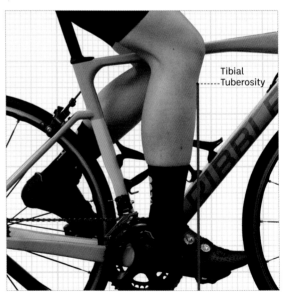

Tibial Tuberosity

Note the difference here in the position of the knee. A vertical line down from the bottom of the knee bisects the pedal spindle, reducing the forces of the patella.

'The Myth of KOPS'). Practically speaking it is hard for some to find the anatomical landmarks accurately, and the plumb line can move, making the vertical judgement subjective. KOPS also has some drawbacks when it comes to speciality riding, for example time trials.

If KOPS is to be used, I like the idea of simply using a straight edge (for example, a metre ruler), placing it in front of the kneecap and making sure this is in front of the pedal spindle. Used in this way, KOPS has helped many riders get themselves into a safe setback position.

Of course, as with all static measuring, the drawback with this method is that it is dependent on the rider sitting exactly where they would be on the saddle while they are riding. This is surprisingly hard to mock up in a clinical environment.

How to set saddle setback – dynamic

The Retül system provides the setback as an average of over 10,000 data points of the knee in relation to the foot over 15 seconds of riding. This gives a clear indication of where the rider's position is while actually riding. Fitters use this data to adjust saddle setback, in this case until the knee is on average more often behind the foot, indicating a safe saddle setback. I know most of us don't have a Retül system sitting in our garage and it's good to remind ourselves that while dynamic

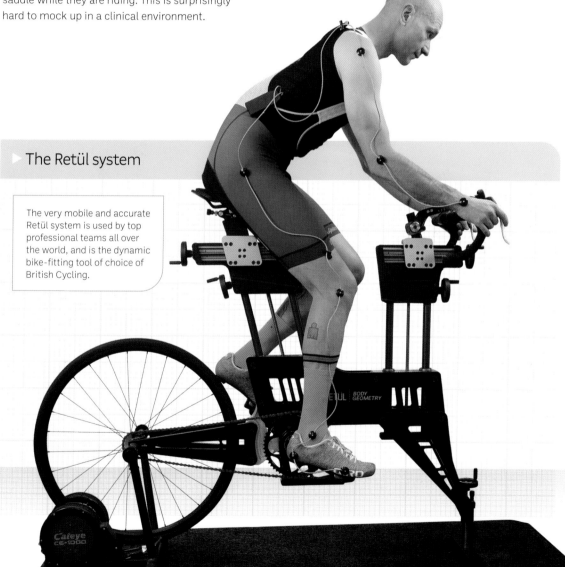

► The Retül system

The very mobile and accurate Retül system is used by top professional teams all over the world, and is the dynamic bike-fitting tool of choice of British Cycling.

measurement systems are the most advanced method of bike fitting, they are still measurement systems – just the same as that metre ruler! The skill is in the interpretation of the data.

The very mobile and accurate Retül system is used by top professional teams all over the world, and is my dynamic bike-fitting tool of choice.

How to set saddle tilt

When I wrote the first edition of this book, if you wanted to compete in a UCI-sanctioned event, you'd have to ride with a completely level saddle. However, because of the research I was involved in looking at how to reduce saddle health issues in riders, the UCI changed this ruling and now allows up to nine degrees of tilt. I'm really proud of having left this legacy in the sport and it is undoubtedly benefiting rider health and well-being.

Those suffering from genital numbness often find huge relief in angling the saddle down a degree or two. The shape of some people's anatomy requires this to help roll the perineum and other tissues out of harm's

way. If we examined most people's saddles they would be level or slightly down. There is no good reason I am aware of to have the nose up – and if I see this I always suggest changing it. A common reason given by those I find with a nose up is that they need to do this to avoid sliding forward on the saddle. This is a classic case of adjusting the wrong fit coordinate: it is more than likely that the saddle height or front/rear balance is incorrect, tipping the rider forward, and it is these issues that need to be corrected, rather than blocking the rider into position by angling the nose of the saddle upwards.

Amateur mountain bikers prefer a slightly nose-down saddle for a simple reason – it stops them catching their shorts every time they sit down from standing on the pedals, which they do a lot more than road riders.

Saddle choice

For some riders, the quest for a comfortable saddle can be frustrating, seemingly endless and expensive. I've had riders turning up to bike fits with a bag of

▶ Different saddle angles

LEVEL OR NOSE DOWN

The angle of the saddle can make a huge difference to a person's fit due to its profound effect on the rotation of the pelvis. I generally recommend the saddle is level or slightly down.

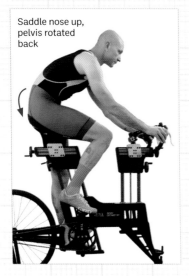

Saddle nose up, pelvis rotated back

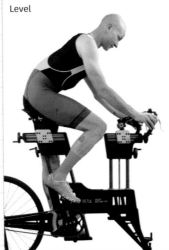

Level

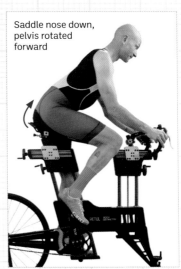

Saddle nose down, pelvis rotated forward

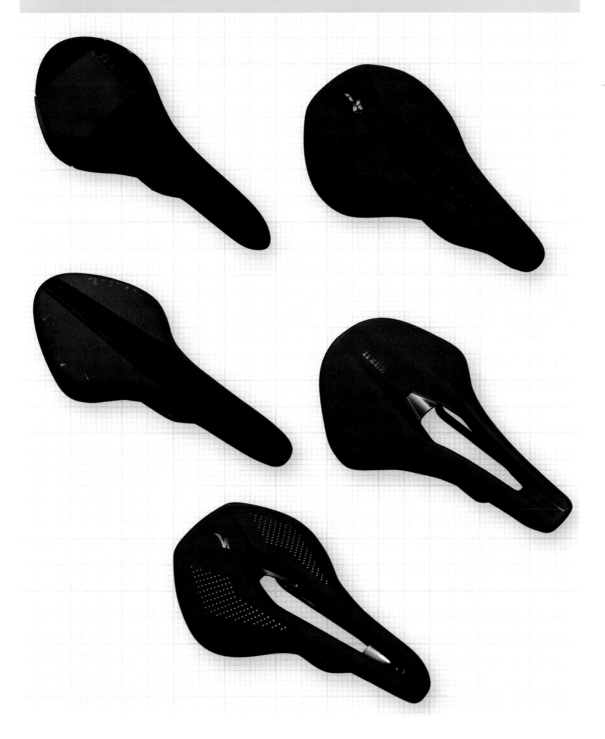

▶ A selection of saddles

10 saddles that they've tried in their search for the perfect perch. I've been involved in the design and construction of saddles for Olympians using various materials, including the silicone rubber used in breast implants. I was the driving force behind a saddle health initiative for female riders on the Great Britain Cycling Team and I'm currently working with saddle manufacturers to develop new designs and products. In short, I've spent an awful lot of time thinking about and dealing with saddles!

Get your position right

Before we start discussing which saddle types might suit you, and definitely before you start spending money on a new one, make sure that you've dialled in your saddle height, fore/aft position and tilt correctly. Refer to the previous advice on saddle position and find the window of fit that is most appropriate to the type of riding you're doing. This is essential, because if a saddle isn't in the right place, it's never going to be comfortable, so don't bin that saddle you've been suffering on – check your position first.

Saddle design

One of the reasons that people get so confused about saddles is simply the huge amount of apparent choice on the market. The bottom line, though (excuse the pun), is that the basic shape of saddles hasn't changed that much from the advent of cycling to now. In fact, when you look at very traditional saddles, such as a Brooks, one of those wouldn't look out of place on a Victorian bike and there are still many riders who swear by these today.

Saddles tend to come in and out of fashion with fairly minor changes in shape, length, flare and the materials used. From those early Brooks-type saddles, we then had a period when the likes of the Selle Italia Flight set the template. The next phase was for longer and narrower saddles, such as the Fizik Arione and Antares, and now we've gone short and stubby with saddles like the Specialized Power.

Variations in saddle shape and design are limited by the role a saddle has to do, our anatomy and by how they are attached to the bike. Double rails atop a seat post are set in stone, from a budget kids' bike through

▶ The same rider's geobimized scans for TT, road and MTB

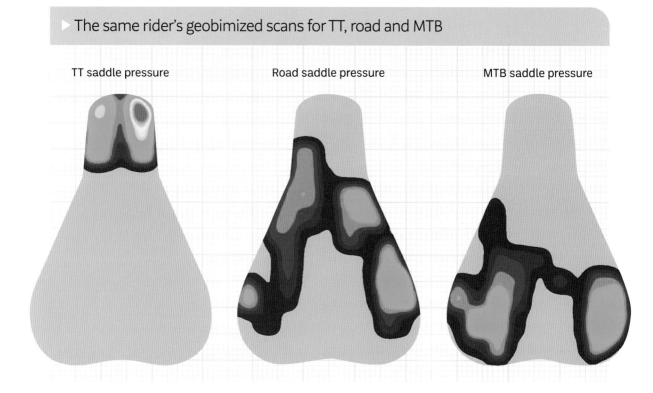

TT saddle pressure

Road saddle pressure

MTB saddle pressure

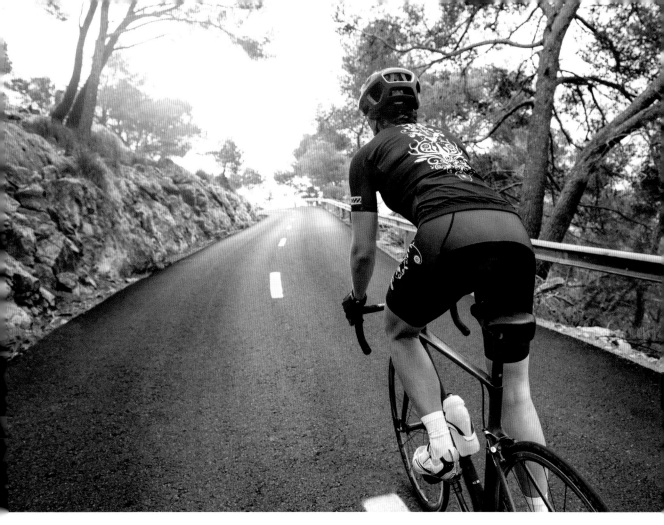

to the highest-tech aero pro bike. If you really wanted to make a difference in saddle design, you'd start from scratch, ditch the rails and maybe look at some sort of mono pin design, but, like a lot of aspects of cycling, change takes a long time.

Not simply trial and error

Once you're certain that your saddle is positioned correctly, a lot of riders then take almost a trial-and-error approach to finding the right saddle. As I've said, I've had riders come to me with upwards of 10 saddles they've tried, probably costing upwards of £100 each, and this can be a costly exercise. So, although there is definitely a fair amount of art and guesswork that go with the science of saddle choice, there are a number of factors to consider that can help you to narrow down your choice.

Type of riding

In the same way that a time trial position is very different to a road, mountain biking or commuting position, so too is how you sit on the saddle for each of those disciplines. You'll often see riders with totally inappropriate saddles for the type of riding they're doing and a simple swap can be revelatory for them.

A great example of this is the number of cyclists I've seen who've put a twin-nosed ISM saddle on a road bike. These saddles are great for aggressive time trial and track positions, where your hips are rotated right forward and you're sat right on the nose of the saddle, but for a road position they rarely work as they're very wide on the nose and just get in the way. Simply looking to see what usage a manufacturer recommends a saddle for can be a great starting point.

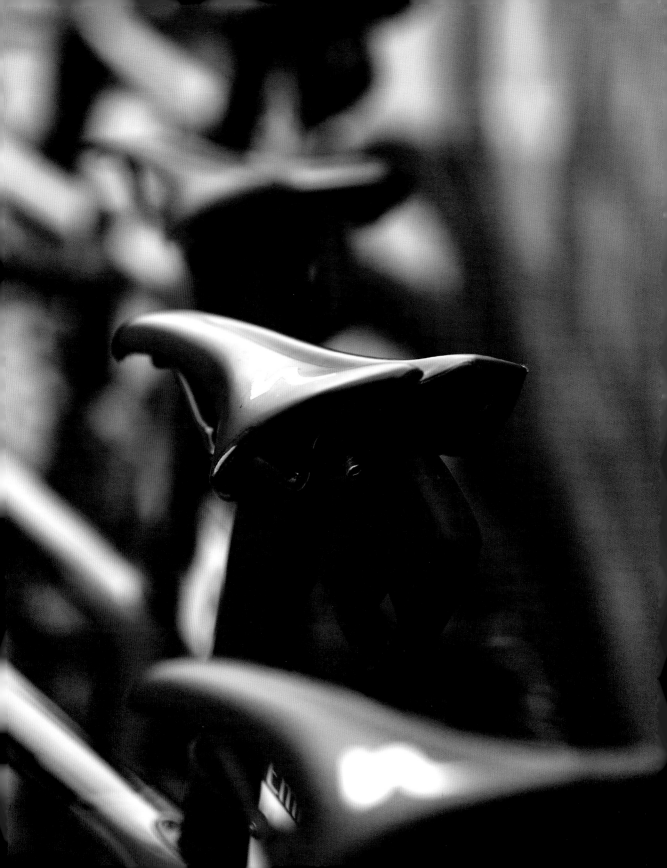

That said, some saddles can be incredibly accommodating and versatile. I know one rider who has a Fizik Arione on every single one of his bikes, from track pursuit through to mountain bike. What's interesting, though, is that the wear patches on each saddle are different. On the pursuit bike it's about an inch on the nose, the road bike slightly further back and, on his mountain bike, it's polished smooth where his sit bones would be and on the wings. This saddle works across all disciplines for him because, first, his position is correct and, second, because it's such a long saddle it allows for a wide range of sitting options.

The opposite can be true of some shorter-nosed saddle designs, especially those that are slightly scooped and hold you fixed in a position. There's very little room for positional error and, although they can be extremely supportive and comfortable if your position is right, if it's off, it's not going to be a comfortable ride. So, again, double-check your saddle positioning.

Saddle width

Once you've identified the type of riding you'll be doing, you then want to consider saddle width and you can get a good idea of this from measuring the distance between your sit bones – ischial tuberosity. This is what happens in a lot of bike shops that offer saddle fitting. They'll get you to sit on a reactive surface, your sit bones will leave an impression and they can then measure the distance between them. In my bike fit lab, I use a digital system, but you can easily replicate this process at home.

Take a piece of aluminium kitchen foil and place it on a carpeted stair. Sit on the foil, lean forward a bit to approximate your riding position, then lift your feet. This should leave a good impression of your rear in the foil, and you can measure between the two points of deepest impression to get your sit bone width. Once you have this distance you can then collate it to saddle width.

The narrowest saddles on the market will be around 138mm, right through to the widest female-specific and leisure saddles, which will be in the 155–165mm range.

Although you can see from the scans, particularly on road and TT set-ups, minimal weight is going through the sit bones and, as all riders get fitter and rotate forward into more aggressive positions, this also applies, it's still a valid gauge for refining your search for your perfect saddle. Although you might not be sitting on your sit bones, the rest of the saddle will be designed and shaped in proportion to this measurement. Women in particular have wider hips and sit bones, so saddles designed for them will accommodate this. It's also worth noting, though, that women's pelvises come together quicker and so, although a saddle might be wider at the rear, it needs to get out of the way quicker so as not to interfere with the pedalling motion. The Specialized Power does this very well.

Saddle length

As I mentioned earlier, a longer saddle, such as a Fizik Arione, gives you the opportunity to move on it, adopt slightly different positions and can accommodate different disciplines. Longer saddles tend to be narrower, though, because to allow the length without impacting on pedal stroke they can't start especially wide.

Much of the early development of short-nosed saddles was to circumvent the UCI ruling that states that the nose of the saddle has to be 5cm behind the centre of the bottom bracket. Infamously Graeme Obree took a hacksaw to his saddle after falling foul of the commissaires and, when they disallowed this too, fitted a saddle from a child's BMX.

Saddle manufacturers started to develop commercial short-nosed saddles, but soon found that there was little interest in them from the pro peloton. The reason for this is that, within a racing season or a stage race, the rider will be making solo breaks, climbing, riding pavé or chilling in the bunch, and all of these require a slightly different position, which makes a longer saddle the road pro's choice. However, they have found that these shorter saddles are incredibly popular with amateur riders. My theory for this is that, if you do get a short-nosed saddle positioned right, you can't help but sit in the right place. Also, because they're often fairly wide, they can give quite a lot of stability and support, which many riders like the feel of. You've also got to remember that in terms of weight distribution pros and stronger riders will be putting far more pressure through their pedals and less on the saddle. For this reason, the support/stability role of the saddle is far less important to them. Finally, for women riders, a short-nosed saddle can be wider at the rear to provide sit bone support, but not interfere with their thigh movement.

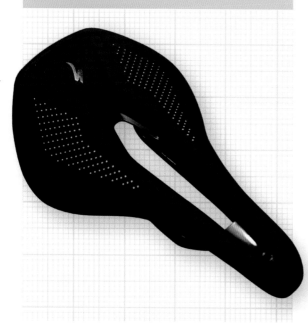

▶ Saddle with cut-out

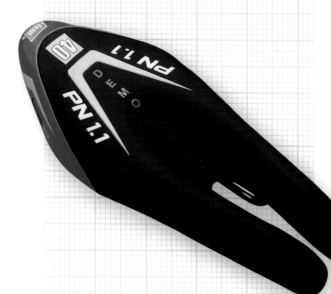

▶ Split-nosed saddle

CUSHIONING

When you're buying a saddle, it's worth remembering that, more often than not the more you spend the less you get. This particularly applies to cushioning as, along with the use of titanium and carbon fibre in the quest for lower weight, superfluous padding is one of the first things to be sacrificed. High-performance saddles are all about minimum weight, maximal stiffness and, remembering what I said about stronger riders putting more pressure through their pedals, not prioritising support and stability.

At the opposite end of the spectrum, you get heavily padded 'leisure saddles', gel covers and saddles on exercise bikes that are more like sofas! Although some riders do undoubtably require more cushioning than others, if you're having to resort to extreme or extra cushioning, it's more than likely that the fundamentals of your saddle position, length and width are incorrect and you're compensating for this. This is why you see such big and heavily padded saddles on commercial exercise bikes, as they're having to accommodate a wide range of users, the majority of whom won't be cyclists and definitely won't have much idea of their riding position.

CUT-OUTS AND CHANNELS

Saddle cut-outs were developed for male cyclists to combat penile numbness which, caused by compression of the dorsal penile nerve, if ignored, can be symptomatic in the development of erectile dysfunction. Excessive pressure can also damage and lead to infections of the urethra. This is characterised by burning or stinging when going to the toilet after a ride or, in severe cases, blood in the urine. Both of these symptoms should be acted on immediately and medical advice sought. Saddles with central cut-outs can help to prevent these conditions.

Many cut-out designs are marketed as female-specific, but in reality are just modified male designs. Trauma and inflammation of the labial tissues is a fairly common issue in female riders. For some women, cut-out designs can be effective, but for others it can just shift the problem or even make it worse. For example, some cut-out saddle designs will alleviate pressure on the inner labia, but can then transfer it to the outer labia instead. If left, the inflammation and swelling can become serious, make the area more prone to further damage and, due to adopting unusual positions on the saddle to try to alleviate the discomfort, can lead to secondary injuries to the back or knees. It's definitely an area where the cycling industry is letting women down and I'm personally pushing for more women-specific saddle choices.

SPLIT-NOSED SADDLES

Split-nosed saddles, such as the ISM, are designed for, and most suited to, aggressive time trial and track positions where the rider's pelvis is rotated forward. Most road riders find them too wide at the nose for more 'sat back' positions.

This width is mainly because of the vigorous testing that saddles have to undergo. Simulated in a test lab, they have to withstand both sudden impacts, as if you were hitting a pothole, and constant high-frequency smaller impacts and vibrations, or road buzz. Split-nosed designs are inherently weaker and, to withstand the testing, there's a limit to how thin they can be.

In a hips-rotated-forward time trial position, you'll be sat right on your pubic rami (a group of bones that make up part of the pelvis), and a split-nose saddle facilitates this, because, as the prongs move slightly as you pedal, it supports the pubic rami very well and the gap provides central pressure relief to sensitive soft tissue areas.

They're an incredibly popular saddle choice among time triallist and triathletes and, at the Ironman World Championships in Kona, Hawaii, you'll see about 50 percent of the field riding them. They do provoke a bit of a love/hate reaction though, and when I was working with the GB women's team pursuit squad it was either love at first ride or 'don't ever come near me with that saddle again'.

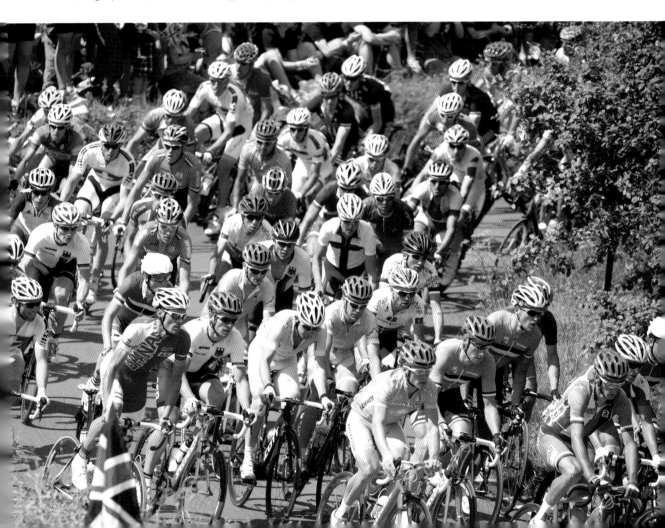

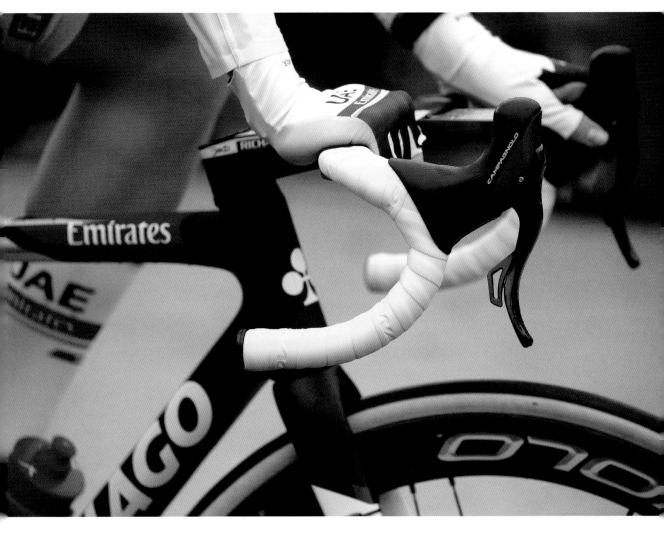

Handlebars

There is a bewildering array of shapes and sizes of handlebars on the market. Width is traditionally the main fit parameter, but the shape and size matter too. It is generally accepted that handlebar width for road riders should be the width of your shoulders. This can be measured on and off the bike. On the bike the lateral side (outside) of the shoulders should be in line with the thumb/index finger on the brake hood. Off the bike, measure between the bony outcrops at the end of the collarbone – the acromia (singular, acromion) as they are known. This again gives a good guide to the appropriate handlebar width.

It's important to get this measure correct as too-wide a hand placement leads to fatigue and numbness in the hands, due to their being splayed out. This also affects handling, making turning the bike slower. Having too-narrow a hand placement can be tiring for the triceps, which have to bear a greater load, and will affect the handling by making the steering quicker and the bike 'twitchier'.

Exceptions to these general rules are mountain bikers who ride with wide handlebars for control reasons and track sprinters who prefer narrower bars to help them manoeuvre – narrower bars mean it is easier for them to get in between riders. Some specialist road sprinters do this as well.

Shape

Most people just ride the bars that a bike comes with. If you need to change them or are having problems with reach, comfort or handling, take the opportunity to consider the shape of the handlebar. In an ideal world, your riding style, hand size and reach should determine this.

The anatomy of a handlebar is shown in the picture on the next page. The horizontal top section is where your hands reside for most of the time when climbing. For this reason climbers often prefer this bit to be wider to give more room for changing the positions of their hands. They will sometimes also prefer an oval or flat top section to optimise hand grip. Track sprinters, on the other hand, will go for a shorter horizontal top section with a rounded curve to the drops to help get the narrower bar mentioned earlier, and to avoid bumping their wrist or forearm against the top section while in the drops.

DROP AND REACH

The drop and reach of a handlebar is an extension of the fit process we described earlier. Obviously the stack and reach of the frame, along with the height and length of the stem, primarily determine drop and reach, but the choice of handlebar can have a subtle influence on the drop and reach within the fit window.

Deep bars with a long reach and big drop are preferred by riders with long arms, as they help them achieve a good, low aero position when in the drops. Riders with a shorter reach generally prefer shorter, shallower handlebars that do not require them to overreach or extend into a deep drop position.

The actual shape of the handlebar drop has changed over the years with some now incorporating a flat section into the curve. These are called anatomical bars. Some riders prefer them, but as with saddles, handlebar variations at this level are down to individual choice and are most likely determined by comfort.

With the increase in popularity of gravel cycling, you're also seeing bars with extreme flare. The theory is that the flare effectively widens the bars when you're on the drops, and so gives more control and stability when descending off-road. However, there is a trade-off with hood angle so ultra wide and flared bars might not suit all.

▶ Measuring handlebar width

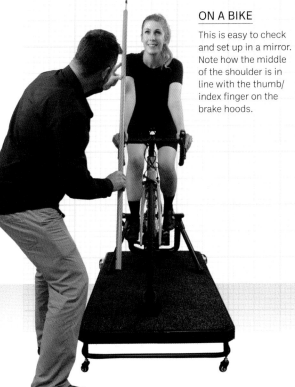

ON A BIKE

This is easy to check and set up in a mirror. Note how the middle of the shoulder is in line with the thumb/index finger on the brake hoods.

OFF THE BIKE

The measure is from acromion to acromion (the pointy bit of bone you can feel where your arm meets your shoulder).

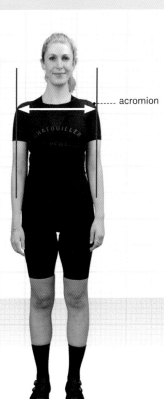

⋯⋯⋯ acromion

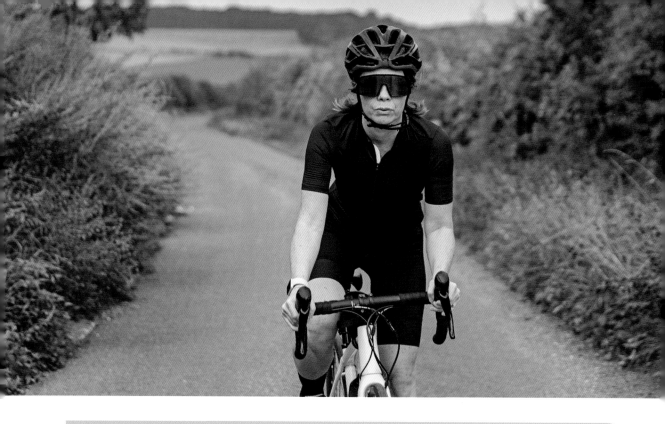

▶ Anatomy of handlebars

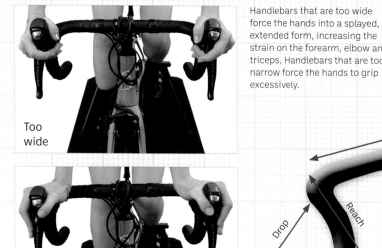

Too
wide

Too
narrow

Handlebars that are too wide
force the hands into a splayed,
extended form, increasing the
strain on the forearm, elbow and
triceps. Handlebars that are too
narrow force the hands to grip
excessively.

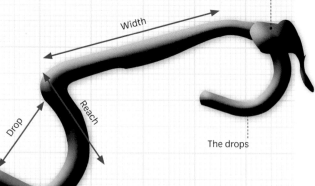

Brake hoods

Width

Drop

Reach

The drops

▶ Different drops

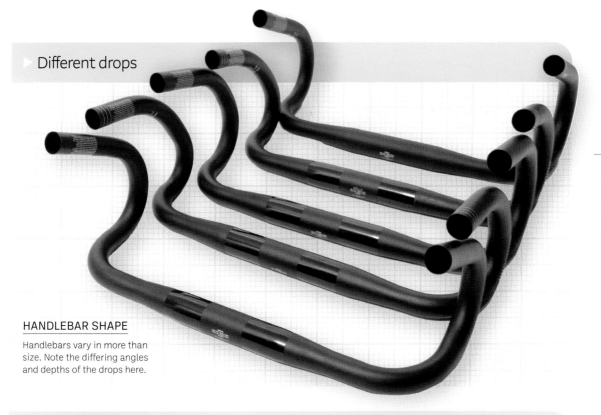

HANDLEBAR SHAPE

Handlebars vary in more than size. Note the differing angles and depths of the drops here.

▶ Flared gravel set-up

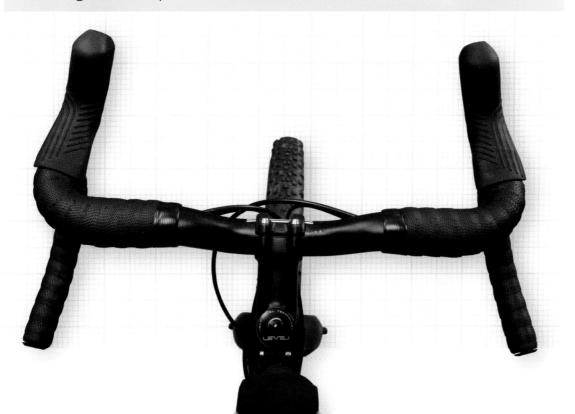

Brake levers

I can't believe how many bike fits I have done where the only thing I have changed is the position of the brake lever and have found that this has solved all the rider's fit issues. The position of the brake lever is crucial and should not be overlooked. The hoods of the brake lever are where most of us rest our hands while riding. The amount of engineering that goes into shaping a Dura Ace or other top-end hood/brake lever makes it the most expensive contact point on the bike – and yet so often we pay little or no attention to its position.

The placing of the brake lever has to allow the rider to access the brakes when their hands are on the hoods and also when they move to the drops. Bike manufacturers work from this premise when designing them, so it makes sense to set them up as intended. A simple method employed by many is to set the tip of the lever in line with the end of the handlebar drop.

If you find that your brake levers are closer to the horizontal top section of the bars and this is where you are comfortable, it may mean that your reach or drop is set up too long or too deep. The brake levers' position in this case is a fit compromise, trying to account for other suboptimal fit coordinates. Shortening or lowering the stem may allow the brake lever to be more correctly positioned.

Mountain bikers are an exception once again. Here the brake levers are set in line with the grip, which is determined by the arm's angle of approach to the bar, normally around 30-40 degrees. This position allows comfortable braking both in and out of the saddle.

HOOD ANGLE

You should be aiming for the flat portion of your hoods to be level or with a slight upward tilt. If you're having to rotate them so they're pointing skywards this suggests possible issues with stack height, reach or both.

Handlebar position

Where the handlebars are positioned, in terms of height and length from the saddle, determines your reach. Sometimes this is referred to as the postural 'length'. It is the most individual part of the bike fit as so many factors contribute to its setting once you have your seat height and setback. Apart from some very basic guidelines it is largely determined by the individual's strength and flexibility through their hamstrings, lower back, thoracic spine, shoulders, neck and arms – nearly the whole body's kinetic chain.

The position of the handlebars not only determines the reach, but also the angle of the torso or back. This measurement provides a useful expression of someone's overall position and reach.

The recommended torso angle for recreational cyclists is 45-55 degrees. This allows a relaxed riding position, typically with little or no saddle-to-bar drop in height and a comfortable reach. Faster road riders have a torso or back angle of anything from 45 to 30 degrees. I describe this as being more aggressive: it's adopted to go faster, race and produce more power.

▶ **Brake lever set-up**

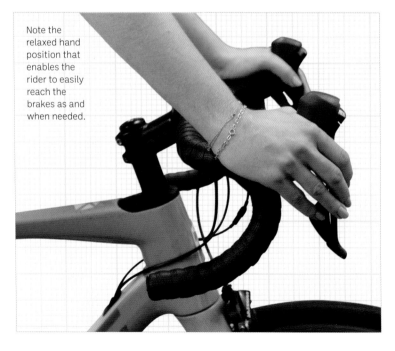

Note the relaxed hand position that enables the rider to easily reach the brakes as and when needed.

► Correct hood angle

► Incorrect hood angle

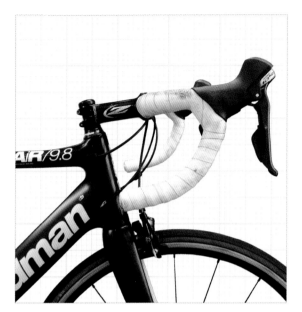

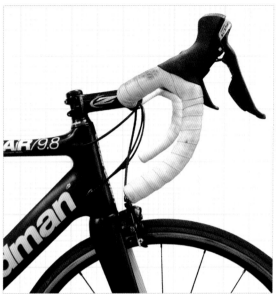

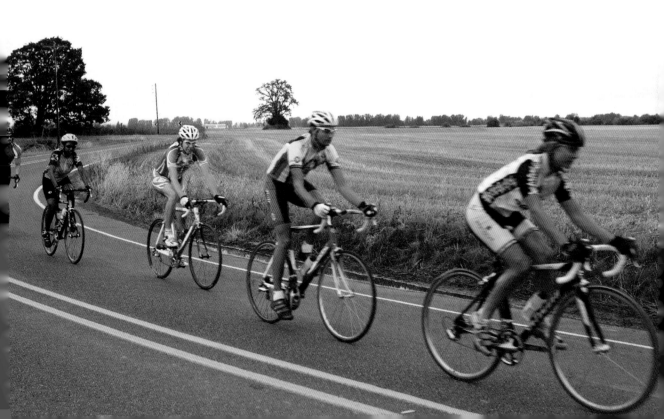

Time triallists are the most aggressive, aiming for a 'flat back' – a torso angle as low as possible to achieve an aerodynamic position. The use of aero bars enables these very low front-end positions to be assumed, but they require great flexibility and a lot of adaptation.

All the factors I've mentioned affecting reach are in turn affected by our age. As we all get stiffer and less adaptable our ability to adopt aggressive positions (at least without a good deal of suffering) wanes.

How to set handlebar height and length-reach

There are some old CONI-style anatomical approximations, the first of which involves putting your elbow against the saddle front and extending your arm and open hand towards the handlebars. Adjust the bar position until only an inch or two of space exists between it and your middle finger. Another method advocates measuring the width of your fist when clenched and sizing your stem to match to achieve the correct reach. As with all of these anatomical approximations, the drawback is that they are limited by a lack of sensitivity to individual characteristics. So once again they may work for some, but not for others – and it's hard to tell who these methods *will* work for.

Various authors (Silberman et al. 2005) make reference to the vertical distance between the saddle and the top of the bars – sometimes termed the saddle-to-bar drop – which should be 1.3 inches (2.5–8cm). None make reference to finding where you should set up within that range. In my experience there are so many factors contributing to an individual's ability to reach forward that it is impossible to apply a simplistic rule of thumb.

It appears so difficult to quantify that some have even suggested the 'balance' method. It's regularly quoted that a rider's weight distribution should be roughly 40-45 per cent on the front end and 55-60 per cent on the back. However, no one has developed an effective way of assessing or measuring this yet, meaning it's so subjective that while balance is important, I don't think you can use it as the primary measure to set reach. Too many components of fit

▶ Different torso positions according to position of handlebars

Good

A

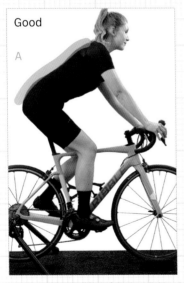

Too long

B

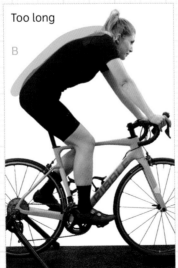

Too short

C

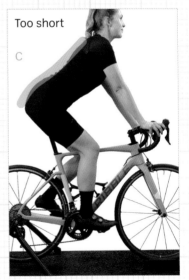

Note how the position of the handlebars in B is too long for the rider, making her stretch her arms and back and crane her neck, and C is too short and has bunched the rider up, making her torso (back angle) too high and putting too much weight on her back end.

contribute to balance, not reach alone.

I advocate using a large amount of common sense and 'feel' to set handlebar reach and height. The most common mistake I see is people setting themselves up in aggressive positions without consideration for their body's ability to hold them for any length of time. They often suffer these positions until they seek help or become injured.

In order to find – and I mean find in the sense of explore – your handlebar's ideal position, start by setting out to achieve the following: with your hands on the hoods or tops your arms should feel relaxed, and you should be able to ride with your elbows slightly bent and feel at ease with this. If the saddle-to-bar drop is too much for you, your arms will straighten and tend to lock out. Relaxing your arms or bending the elbows will feel difficult as there will be too much weight on the arms, meaning your hands will often become numb or tingling quickly in one position. You should also be able to look up the road while cycling easily without feeling strain or pain in your neck or in between your shoulder blades.

Set your handlebars to the above parameters first, and don't be ashamed if you have a high front end: it's like that for a reason if the above guidelines have been obeyed, because it's all your body will allow for now. We can all work on our flexibility to a point and, indeed, the very nature of riding a bike helps us adapt to this particular body position. An aggressive position should be evolved over time by slowly nudging the handlebar height down or extending your stem. Remember: the bike is adjustable, the rider is adaptable. One takes seconds, the other for most of us unfortunately takes a lot longer!

Pedals

The history of cycling pedals is long and rich. Today we have many different types of pedal, from platform pedals, where your foot is free to make whatever contact you wish and clips can be added to help position the foot more rigidly, to clipless pedals with cleats that lock your cycling shoe into your pedal. The advantage of cleats is that more of your force and

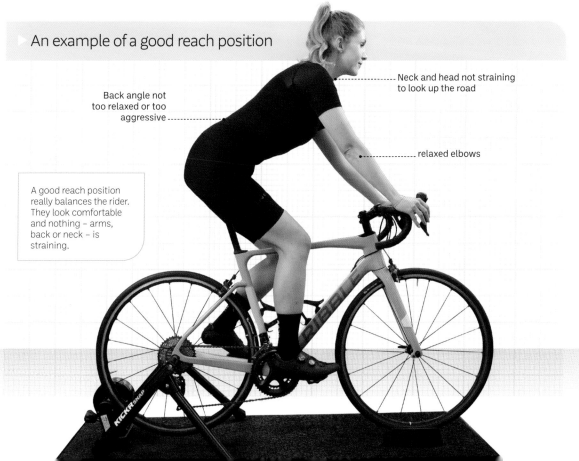

▶ An example of a good reach position

Back angle not too relaxed or too aggressive ·············

Neck and head not straining to look up the road

relaxed elbows

A good reach position really balances the rider. They look comfortable and nothing – arms, back or neck – is straining.

▶ The bike is adjustable and the rider is adaptable

Note the aggressive road position and even more agressive time trial postion. It takes time to adapt to these for the best of us, and unfortunately some of us need to accept that we are not adaptable enough.

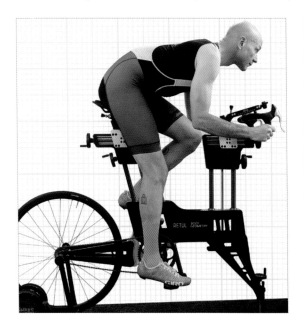
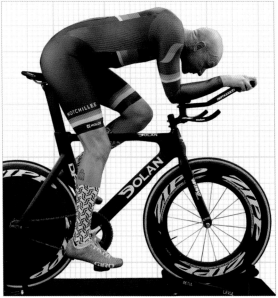

▶ Different stem lengths and their impact on handling the bike

At the extremes of stem length the handling of a bike can be affected, some argue, due to the relative position of the hands on the handlebar behind, or in front of, the front wheel hub. Too short a stem and handling can become twitchy, too long and handling is laboured.

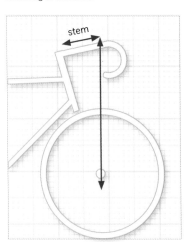
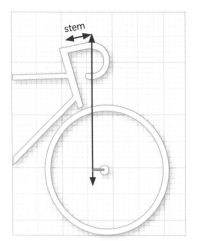
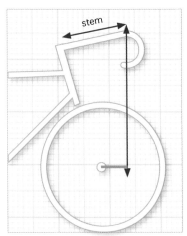

drive is applied directly and there is less energy or force wasted controlling your foot's position on the pedal. The extent of the cleat's locking is itself variable, from mountain bike pedals that allow you to disengage at the slightest sign that you need to, to the incredible tensioned cleats used by track sprinters to prevent them pulling their feet out of the pedal during a standing start.

The transition from free to clipless (cleated) is what most people struggle with. It takes time to get used to riding when locked into the pedal and therefore onto the bike. I recommend practising somewhere safe for as long as is necessary before venturing out onto busy roads or mountain bike trails where the ability to exit the pedal is vital.

The million dollar question is: which clipless pedal is right for me? As usual, there isn't a simple answer. Pedal choice – like that of saddle – is largely down to personal preference and what works for an individual rider. The main brands are well represented across

Knock-on effect on handling

If in setting your handlebars up you have noticed a change in the bike's handling, a slight alteration is to be expected. If your bike frame size is correct a stem length of between 10–12cm should be normal. Less or more than this tends to change the handling of a road bike as your weight is either too far forward or is behind the hub of the front wheel. I accept 10-14cm stem lengths with professional riders, but stems that achieve a comfortable reach at below 10cm or beyond 14cm probably indicate the frame size of the bike is less than optimal for you (see page 77 for more on frame size).

the riders I see and it largely comes down to personal choice, but here are some guidelines.

When you make your choice, consider the adjustments a pedal system offers. The section on float (the amount of movement a cleat allows – see page 72) underlines the importance of the set-up of the pedal/foot interaction. If you have a history of knee pain, make sure the pedal system you choose has the adjustability you need to accommodate your biomechanics. Some of us will happily slip into a fixed clipless pedal with no float and spend little time

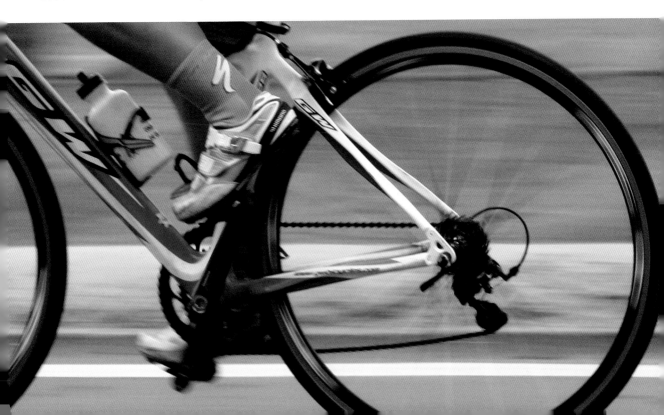

setting them up and never have a problem (these are the macro-absorbers among us!). The rest, on a sliding scale, need to spend a bit more time working out what degree of fixing we can accept, given that ours is a sport of repetitive movement. At the far end of the spectrum, I have found that using Speedplay pedals can help riders who have trouble with their pedal/foot set-up. This is due to their high degree of adjustability – for example, longer spindles for a stance that suits the legs being further apart. For some riders on the road using mountain bike pedals is a good staging post. They are easy to disengage from and are less restricted, making it a good transition before taking on stronger clipless pedals. For some, previous injury history or biomechanics might mean they will keep using mountain bike pedals on a permanent basis.

It's handy to note that the type of 'float' certain pedals allow differs. Float is the allowance for slight rotational movement of the cleat/shoe on the pedal. Look and Shimano pedals have toe float, the rotation being centred at the front of the foot. Speedplay, on the other hand have float centred on the ball of the foot. Some pedal systems have a spring tension that returns the cleat to the central position at the moment in the pedal cycle that the foot allows it to do so, others do not. This tension can cause issues for people unable to control it, in particular knee pain and ITB tightness.

During my time at British Cycling and Team Sky, I suddenly found myself inundated with a spate of knee complaints. Riders who had never before suffered with the issue were complaining and the micro-adjusters were just plain unhappy. After a week or so it all settled down. A common element threaded through those affected – they were all riding a new make of pedals. We asked them if anything had changed at all and just one thing had: the amount of spring tension had been increased. Just one small change like that had affected so many – it shows how sensitive we can be to change.

Foot/pedal interface

The final piece of the puzzle is setting up your foot/pedal interface or, in other words, getting your cleats in the right place on your shoes.

If you are not using a clipless pedal system, you do not need to worry about this section. Your feet will find their own happy place on a flat pedal. However, if you are using the modern clipless pedal this section needs careful attention. Cycling is a sport of repetition and the average cyclist makes 80 revolutions per minute – that's 5,400 revolutions an hour. Which position you choose to lock your foot in – and thereby knee and

Clipless pedals and cleats help you pull up and utilise your hip flexors – or do they?

No, they don't, unless you are a track sprinter and then only really if you're going from a standing start. The work of Barratt and Martin demonstrates clearly that the negative torque seen in most people's upstroke is non-mechanical in nature. This is important to realise as a number of coaches view the negative torque as something that can be addressed by somehow training the hip flexors to pull up more. This cannot be achieved. As stated, the negative torque is non-mechanical in nature – and is created by the weight of the limb on the return of the pedal to TDC slowing the pedal down. The hip flexors work merely to try and get the limb out of the way as quickly as possible. Why?

The overwhelming power being produced on the other pedal by the thigh and glutei extending completely negates any contribution the relatively tiny and biomechanically disadvantaged hip flexor can make.

Warning: with this in mind, the use of decoupled or independent cranks, where you have to return the pedal to TDC using the hip flexor with no assistance from the opposite crank, should be done with caution. With questionable benefit to pedalling force production, these training devices, in my opinion, add to the likelihood of developing tight and dysfunctional hip flexors due to the increased workload demanded in the closed hip position.

therefore whole lower limb – to the pedal is a big deal. It's the flip side of being locked into the bike and able to apply as much possible power to the pedal without wasting energy trying to stabilise the foot/pedal interface. If you are locked in incorrectly, you are open to any number of potential overuse injuries.

Fore/aft

The generally accepted rule of thumb for fore/aft positioning of the cleat is to align the ball of the foot with the centre line of the pedal axle (spindle) in the 3 o'clock position. The ball of the foot (the first head of the metatarsal joint) is the big bony protrusion just behind the big toe. This is where people commonly get bunions. Traditionally, this has been placed over the pedal spindle as it provides the largest contact area of the foot directly above the pedal's axis of rotation, and therefore maximises the biomechanical advantages of the foot to produce optimal power output.

Andy Pruitt suggests that this approach really only works for size 9 US men's feet (UK size 8), as larger feet need more stability, requiring the cleat to be slightly behind the pedal spindle. For smaller feet the opposite applies. Some even advocate using the second and third metatarsals, and Sanderson et al. (1994) suggest the fifth metatarsal head is the anatomical landmark to set fore/aft to. However good the reasoning behind their arguments for this, these landmarks are hard for the non-professional cyclist to find accurately on their own.

I like Todd Carver's take on cleat fore/aft, which is a compromise of all the above and in my experience

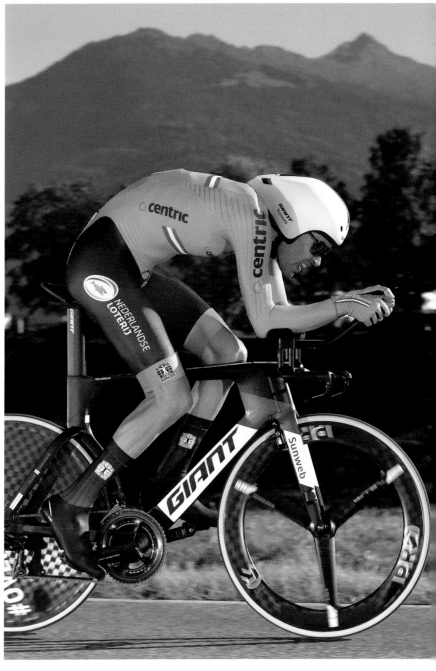

works very well. Find the head of the first metatarsal (ball of the foot). Then find the fifth metatarsal head (if you run your fingers down the outside of your foot, it's the first large bony protrusion you come to). Align the pedal spindle so it bisects the first and fifth metatarsal heads. I find this method helps account for the sizing issue Pruitt highlights and generally gets people into the fit window.

Alterations can be made to this fore/aft position for numerous conditions (see pages 93–94), but the correct positioning of the pedal fore/aft is important for a number of reasons. A forward positioned cleat (so the foot is further back) results in a more up and down movement of the heel as it pivots around a longer lever arm and can produce Achilles issues. It also affects the overall bike set-up by changing the relative position of the foot in relation to the knee (see page 106).

A rearward positioned cleat (so the foot is further forward) helps spread the pressure created when pedalling over more of the foot, and specifically the mid-foot – this can help people reduce forefoot pain (often termed 'hot foot').

For riders who are duck-footed (walking toes out, heels in), moving the cleat rearward can help limit the amount of crank/heel contact.

Having said all this, the jury is out on the potential performance benefits of cleat position.

Many studies have tried to examine the effect on the amount of energy expended with regard to fore/aft cleat position, with inconclusive results. You can find many an internet forum or blog advocating arch or mid-foot cleat position for the most efficient power transfer from the lower limb to the pedal. The simple argument is that by shortening the lever arm of the foot/ankle pedal/cleat interaction you adopt a position that is biomechanically more advantageous for the transfer of power. To date research in this area has been limited.

Rotation

Back in the 1970s, the CONI manual advocated everyone adopting a very pigeon-toed (heels out, toes in) riding style, with the knees coming into the top tube. If followed slavishly for years, this style could end many cycling careers, or at least reduce many people's enjoyment of cycling.

The rotation, or the angle the cleats are set up at, is important because it is a reflection of each of our

▶ Cleat position

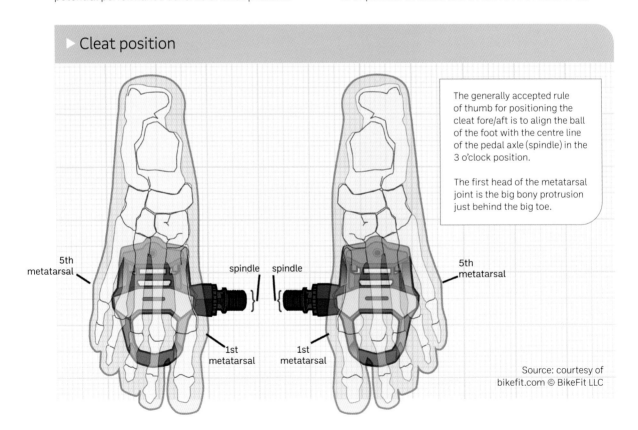

5th metatarsal

spindle spindle

1st metatarsal

1st metatarsal

5th metatarsal

The generally accepted rule of thumb for positioning the cleat fore/aft is to align the ball of the foot with the centre line of the pedal axle (spindle) in the 3 o'clock position.

The first head of the metatarsal joint is the big bony protrusion just behind the big toe.

Source: courtesy of bikefit.com © BikeFit LLC

individual physiques. Have a look at the next 20 or so people who walk past you. Make a mental note of whether they walk with their feet straight ahead (toes/heel in line), like a duck (toes out/heels in) or like a pigeon (toes in/heels out).

If we followed the CONI guidelines only the pigeon-toed among us would be happy. The rest would soon develop overuse injuries such as iliotibial band (ITB) tightness or patello-femoral (kneecap) pain. We should instead set our cleats up to accommodate our natural and unique lower limb biomechanics. If we don't do this, our feet cannot drop the heel in, or 'pronate', as they ought to, meaning that the forces which are usually dispersed by this movement are transferred up the kinetic chain. The weakest point
– usually the knee – will eventually break down.

With fixed cleat/pedal systems (without float), set-up is crucial. With pedal systems that allow rotation/float it is less important, but the midpoint of the rotation/float still needs lining up correctly to gain maximum benefit.

If a rider walks with toes pointing straight ahead they should set their pedals/cleats up so that this is the case on the bike.

If a rider walks with toes out and heels in then they should again set their pedal/cleats up to allow the heels to drop in when they pedal. This subgroup often find they have to move their cleats towards the inside of the shoe to effectively increase the stance width and stop their heels making contact with the crank arm. Some riders drop their heels in so much they often require longer pedal spindles to increase their stance width enough to stop the crank from rubbing.

A pigeon-toed rider needs to make their pedal/cleat system reflect this and have their heels pointing slightly outwards. This subgroup is small in my experience and care should be taken adopting this set-up as it will lead to ITB tightness and irritation in all but those whose biomechanics make it necessary.

▶ Alignment of pedal spindle in relation to first and fifth metatarsal heads

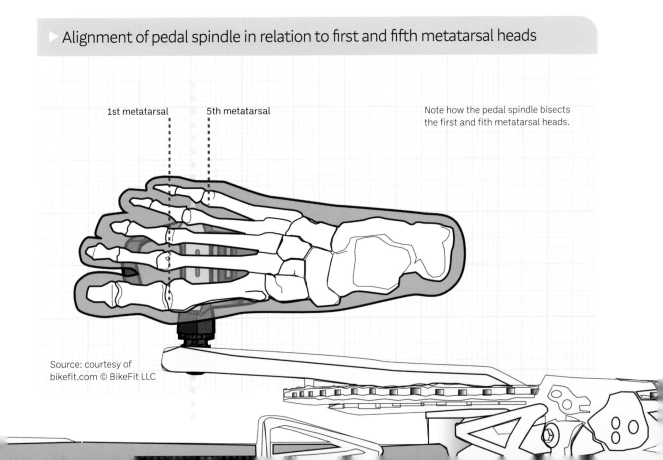

1st metatarsal   5th metatarsal

Note how the pedal spindle bisects the first and fifth metatarsal heads.

Source: courtesy of bikefit.com © BikeFit LLC

Foot/pedal float

As mentioned, 'float' is the small amount of rotational movement the cleat will allow so as not to leave the foot fixed too rigidly to the pedal. In the days when people just pedalled around in old-style toe clips on flat pedals, float existed by accident. In this free-pedal system people's feet were free to migrate to whatever position they needed to.

With the advent of clipless pedal systems in the 1970s, initially all degrees of float were removed. The idea for the locked-in pedal/cleat/shoe system came from ski-boot binding systems. The company Look first made these long before they were a major cycling pedal manufacturer. There was no need for float in skiing so early locking pedal systems offered none. However it wasn't long before cyclists started to experience overuse injuries from being locked into one position. With the cleats set straight ahead as was recommended (and aesthetically pleasing), many riders developed ITB tightness and patello-femoral issues.

The reason for this is that the knee isn't simply a

Changing your set-up

If you have ridden a lot on a certain bike and pedal system, be careful when changing to a new or different set-up. I see many people who have ended up with an injury or pain without knowing that the cause is a change of equipment. For example, when swapping cleats you should take a photo of the old position before removing each one. That way you will be able to get the new ones spot on. I always recommend keeping old shoes and cleats until any new set-up has been tried out over many rides, so that if there is a problem we not only have something to look at in order to establish the cause, we also have the old set-up to ride on until the issue is resolved.

hinge joint, flexing and extending: it twists as well. As we push down on the pedal, the tibia rotates on the femur. Associative rotation and pronation of the foot/

▶ Straight walking style

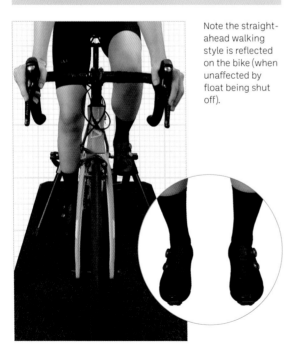

Note the straight-ahead walking style is reflected on the bike (when unaffected by float being shut off).

▶ Duck-footed walking style

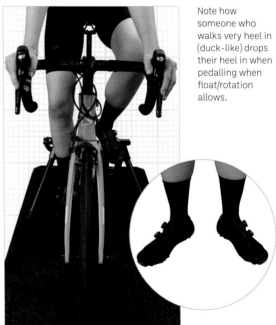

Note how someone who walks very heel in (duck-like) drops their heel in when pedalling when float/rotation allows.

ankle complex occur concurrently. The fixed position of the locked-in clipless pedal system significantly reduces the degrees of motion available for this to occur, resulting in more overuse injuries seen in riders who do not use float than in those who do.

Maury Hull (Ruby and Hull 1993) has done some of the most extensive and scientifically reliable research into the effect of the foot/pedal interface on loading at the knee. The conclusions from his extensive work include the fact that allowing one degree of freedom in float decreases knee-joint loads significantly. He astonished audiences of bike fit professionals at the 2007 SICI conference when he revealed his research findings suggesting that a valgus (inward) not varus (outward) forefoot posting reduced injury forces at the knee joint.

Old myths around float still resonate in the cycling world. Many argue that float requires more 'accessory muscle stabilisation', that is, a lot of effort just stabilising the foot on the pedal (cycling on Speedplay pedals for the first few times feels like pedalling on an ice cube), and is therefore less economical and reduces power. Equally, some argue that float shares or spreads the repetitive loads that stress the knee and surrounding soft tissues. Both camps are wide of the mark in my opinion. The way in which float permits a rider to adopt the biomechanical patterning optimal for their muscles and joints must surely allow them to generate more power than is lost by trying to stabilise in compensation for a few degrees of float – if indeed they have to do that at all.

> Interestingly, track sprint cyclists use floatless locked-in pedal systems extensively and will usually double-up with straps too. However, they do not suffer overuse issues, as the time spent intensely pedalling with restricted movement is usually short. For them the most important thing is that their feet do not unclip when they are starting (for example in a team sprint) or making an extreme acceleration in a match sprint, and removing float helps in this area.

▶ Pigeon-toed walking style

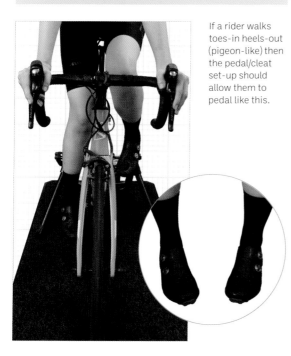

If a rider walks toes-in heels-out (pigeon-like) then the pedal/cleat set-up should allow them to pedal like this.

▶ Heel hitting crank arm

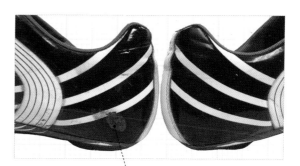

Heel rub: duck-footed rider needs stance-width correction.

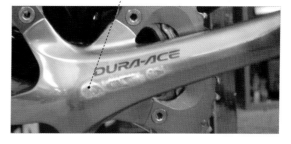

At the same time experience tells me that, while the idea of sharing the load sounds like a persuasive theory, it probably isn't the reason float works. This is because riders who move to a clipless pedal system with adjustable float (such as Speedplay Zeros), usually start with the maximum degree of float available and over time dial the float in, removing what they don't need. The float allows them to find the position they are most happy in on the pedal and then the few degrees remaining after they have removed the extraneous float will allow natural biomechanical lower limb patterning to take place.

Foot pedal side to side

The side-to-side position of the cleats, in terms of how far left or right they sit on the shoe, affects the effective stance width of the bike; that is, the distance between your feet. By positioning the cleat towards the outside or the inside of the shoe you position the foot closer to, or further away from, the crank arm. Hence people with narrow hips trying to align hip/knee/foot may well move their cleats to the outside of their shoes, therefore narrowing their stance and helping to align the hips with the knee and foot. Wider-hipped riders will employ the opposite to gain alignment.

Different pedals offer different amounts of adjustability when it comes to stance width. Speedplay have up to 4mm either side of centre making a total 8mm of adjustability. Some pedal systems offer different sized pedal spindles to people wanting to optimise their stance width. Speedplay offer four different sizes of spindle, for example, and other manufacturers make longer spindle widths for the pro riders in the peloton (the group of riders bunched together in a race), although these are not available commercially.

Stance width

Of all the parameters that are adjustable on a bike, stance width is the most overlooked in my opinion. Until relatively recently, stance width was pretty much set by the width of the bottom bracket on the bike because pedal spindles were almost universally the

---

▶ Toe float varus

TOE FLOAT VS CENTRED FLOAT AND SPRING-CENTRED PEDALS

Most of the pedal systems available use cleat systems that lock in from the front of the shoe. In other words, the float is centred at the front or toe end of the cleat. Speedplay pedals provide centred rotation (see the illustration).

A lot of the pedal systems also employ springs that return the cleat and shoe to the middle position where possible – Shimano Dura Ace, for example. Others use friction that increases as it gets further from the midline. Both give the sensation of centring the foot on the pedal when the forces allow it. When one famous company changed the springs in their top-end pedal to a higher resistance without telling anyone we noticed a sharp spike in knee niggles and pain, as the system had effectively locked down the position if the rider wasn't strong enough to overcome the stronger spring.

Source: courtesy of bikefit.com © BikeFit LLC

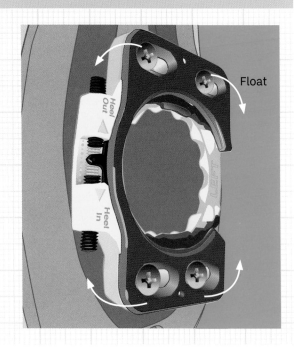

▶ Stance width

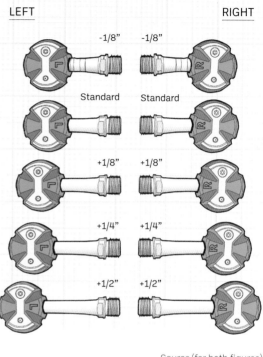

Q angle

Stance width

▶ Different spindle widths

LEFT   RIGHT

-1/8"   -1/8"

Standard   Standard

+1/8"   +1/8"

+1/4"   +1/4"

+1/2"   +1/2"

Source (for both figures):
courtesy of bikefit.com
© BikeFit LLC

same length. This one-size-fits-all approach has always baffled me. People's pelvises, and therefore hip widths, are obviously different – and achieving a hip/knee/foot alignment that delivers a Q angle a rider can cope with is obviously dependent on stance width.

You can see this if you ask someone to perform a squat or a leg press: the foot position that people instinctively adopt on the floor or footplate will vary massively. It's important to bear this in mind if you ride a range of different types of bikes. The bottom bracket widths, and therefore stance widths, will be very different between a road and mountain bike, for example, and even more if you're looking at dedicated indoor bikes and e-Bikes.

Q factor and Q angle

The terms Q factor and Q angle are confusing because they are often used interchangeably. Q angle in cycling refers to the angle formed by the quadriceps as it meets the patella tendon. In general, women have a larger Q angle than men due to having wider hips. Q factor is the distance between the two pedal cranks, which is a measure of stance width and therefore affects the Q angle. I have decided to use the term stance width instead of Q factor to avoid this confusion. I've found that manipulation of the Q angle through stance width has resolved many riders' knee issues.

So what frame size am I?

Despite all of what I've just said about the complications of bike fit and sizing, some of you will still be asking this question. We have discussed the shortcomings of various quick methods – formulae and the like – but I understand many of you won't want to drop £200–300 on a dynamic bike fit, which is the easy answer. The best way to find your frame size cheaply is to not rely on any one single measure. If you're outside the middle area of normal distribution, as discussed earlier, you could end up in trouble. So line up lots of evidence for what frame size you're likely to be and you will have a better chance of getting it right.

I would suggest you do all of these to increase the chances of success:

1 Check with the manufacturer. If you know the make of bike you want, check online. Many manufacturers have websites that give you a guide as to what size you may be. The simplest being your height related to the top tube length. For example, I'm 6'4" tall, and for this height most would recommend a 60cm top tube size bike. Others go into more depth.

2 Use the LeMond method. Measure your inseam and multiple by 0.833 to give you a saddle height. If you take this information to a bike shop they will be able to work out which size frame you need.

3 Use online sizing apps. Many have sprung up, some linked to major manufacturers, and they normally involve measuring a few body parts. For instance, at the time of writing, the ebicycles.com site has a good Road Bike Size Calculator.

4 If you have a bike already, measure that – saddle height and reach and drop. This info will help to place you on the right frame.

Remember, this is sizing, not fitting. Sizing is working out what size bike should work for you, whereas fitting is just that – fitting the bike to you.

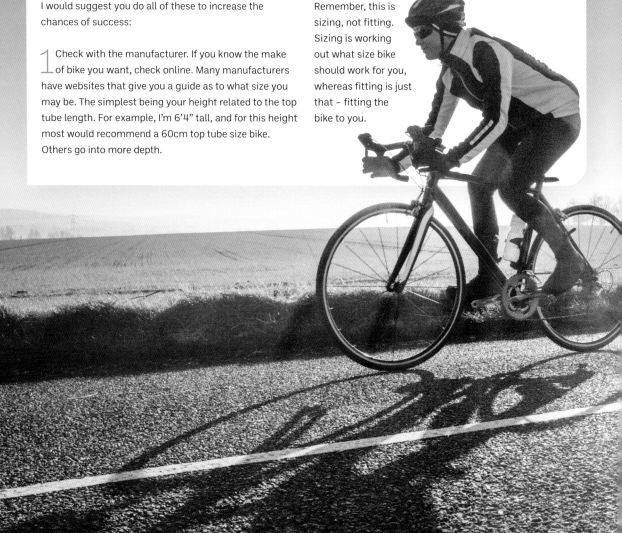

▶ Retűl recommended normal ranges

MEASUREMENT TITLE	NOTES	ROAD	MTB	TT	TRI
Knee angle flexion	–	108°-112°	110°-115°	110°-115°	110°-115°
Knee angle extension	–	35°-40°	35°-40°	37°-42°	37°-42°
Back angle	on hoods for road	45°	50°	20°	25°
Armpit angle to elbow	–	–	–	75°-80°	70°-75°
Armpit angle to wrist	–	90°	75°-80°	–	–
Elbow angle	–	150°-170°	150°-170°	90°-100°	90°-100°
Forearm angle	–	–	–	varies	varies
Ankling range	–	15°-30°	15°-30°	15°-30°	15°-30°
Ankle angle max (plantar flexion)	near top of pedal stroke	95°-105°	95°-105°	95°-105°	95°-105°
Ankle angle min (dorsi flexion)	near bottom of pedal stoke	70°-80°	70°-80°	70°-80°	70°-80°
Hip angle closed	look for bilateral differences	55°-65°	60°-80°	35°-45°	45°-55°
Hip angle open	look for crank length too	-	-	-	-
Knee forward of foot	–	(-10) – 0mm	(-20) – (-10)mm	(+50) – (+100)mm	(+50) – (+100)mm
Hip vertical travel	–	40-60mm	40-60mm	40-60mm	40-60mm

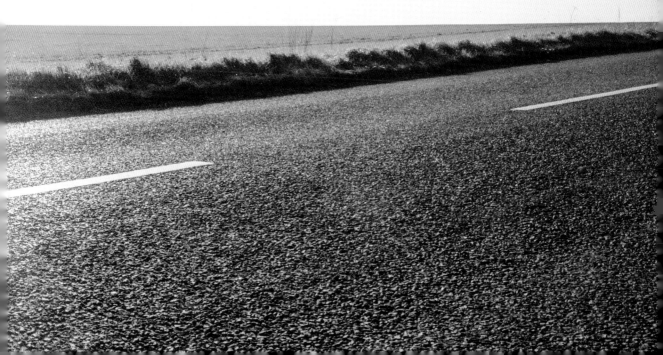

The bike fit detective

Bike fit is undeniably a science, but there's also a fair amount of artistry, intuition and some detective work involved. There are a few common pointers that I regularly see that are strong indicators that something might need tweaking.

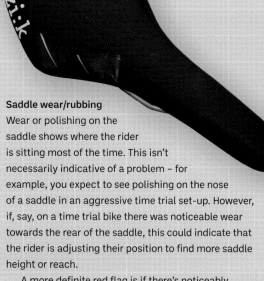

Shoe rub
Rubbing or scuffing on the inside heel region of the shoe can indicate an issue with stance width and/or cleat set-up (either lateral positioning or rotation).

Crank rub
This is what is rubbing against the shoe and, if both marks are present, you definitely know something is up. Possible causes are the same as shoe rub.

Saddle wear/rubbing
Wear or polishing on the saddle shows where the rider is sitting most of the time. This isn't necessarily indicative of a problem – for example, you expect to see polishing on the nose of a saddle in an aggressive time trial set-up. However, if, say, on a time trial bike there was noticeable wear towards the rear of the saddle, this could indicate that the rider is adjusting their position to find more saddle height or reach.

A more definite red flag is if there's noticeably more wear on one side of a saddle than the other. I've even had riders come for a fit with a saddle that they hadn't noticed had effectively collapsed on one side. Such uneven wear could be an indicator of a leg length discrepancy or another similar imbalance.

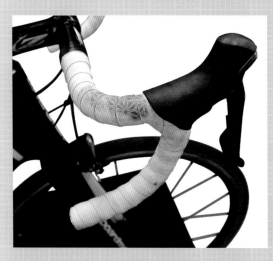

Bar tape wear/marking
By looking at a rider's bar tape, especially if they've been considerate enough to use white tape, it's easy to see where their hands are when riding most of the time. If most of the wear is on the tops, with very little around the hoods or on the drops, either they're spending a lot of time climbing or it's possible that reach might be too long or stack height too low. Similarly, if you see significant wear just back from the hoods, this can suggest that reach is slightly too long or that the hoods aren't correctly set up to offer a comfortable hand position.

Uneven chamois/pad wear
Often before a saddle starts to show uneven wear, a rider's pad can be a really useful early warning system. Again, more wear on one side than the other can be a strong pointer of some form of imbalance.

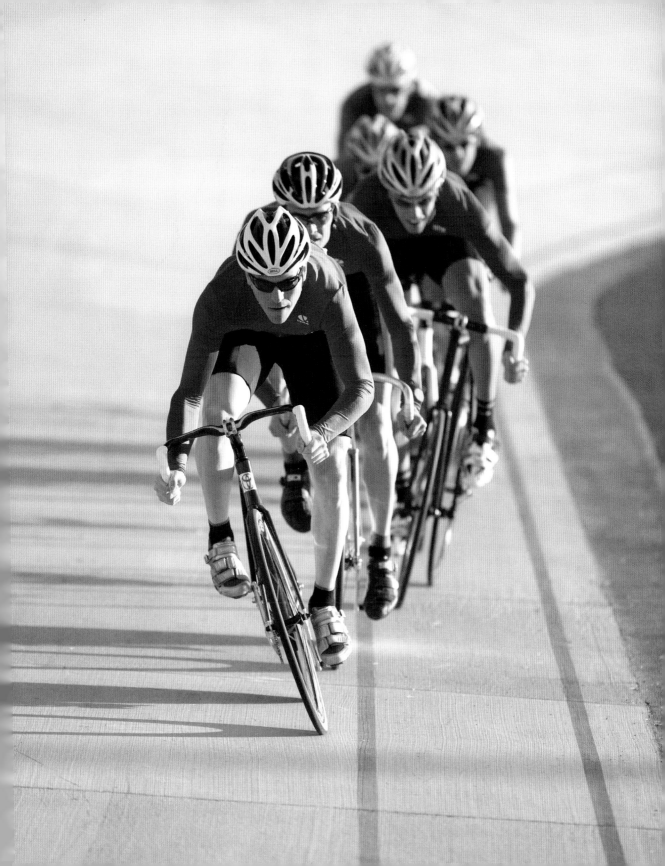

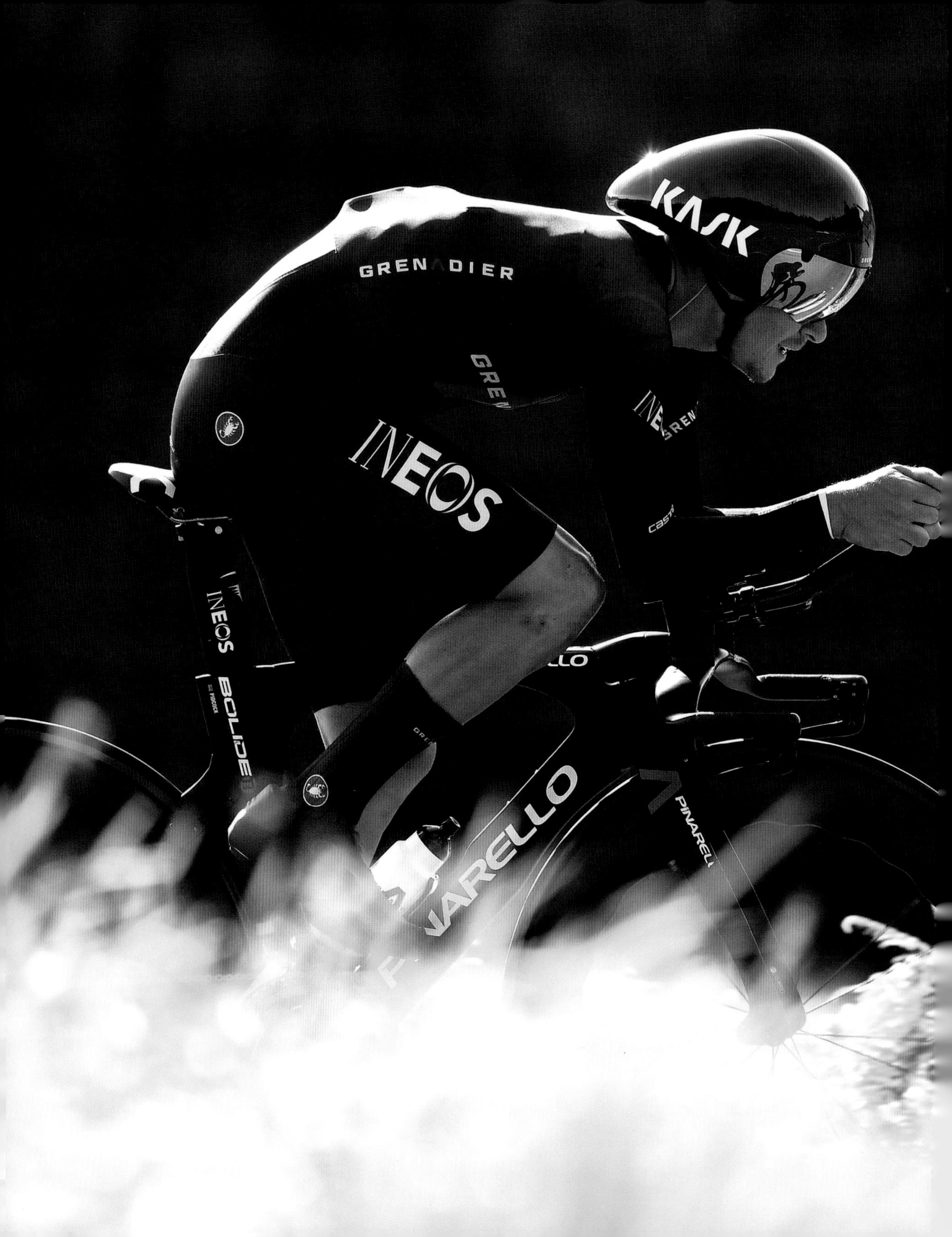

04

The three pillars of fit

The three pillars of fit

To get the right bike fit for you, it is vital to return to first principles. You need to set your goal first. It's not enough to say, 'Just get me the right position on the bike.' The question, as I often say, is: 'For what?'

The right position to cycle down to the shops for five minutes is not the same as to cycle for eight hours on the Étape du Tour. Neither would you attempt to hold Bradley Wiggins's super-aero flat-backed time trial position for a Sunday afternoon ride with the kids.

I like to use this concept to help people understand the balancing act that is a good bike position. It was initially put to me by Chris Boardman on one of the long dark days in the wind tunnel preparing for the London 2012 Olympics. Since then I've adapted it a little.

Imagine three pillars: one made for aerodynamics, one for comfort and one for power. The taller the pillar, the more important the factor is to fit to, but as one pillar goes up, one or both of the others must go down to compensate.

Team pursuit

The first diagram here describes the Olympic Team pursuit position. It could be described as extreme, because it is dictated by only two factors: how aerodynamic and powerful the position is. The time spent in the position is less than four minutes, so comfort pales into insignificance.

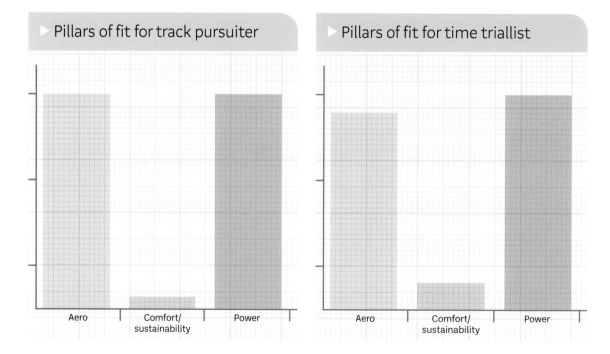

▶ Pillars of fit for track pursuiter

Aero | Comfort/sustainability | Power

▶ Pillars of fit for time triallist

Aero | Comfort/sustainability | Power

Time trial

Most cyclists cannot tolerate the pursuit position much beyond the duration of the event. Exceptions exist – Brad Wiggins's pursuit position is very similar to his Tour de France time-trial position. But he is a special individual who has evolved his position over years and years. Most other cyclists need the comfort factor to be taken into consideration. This is because there is no point being incredibly aero and powerful for four minutes at a time doing a 40-minute time trial. If the position isn't relatively sustainable then all the benefits are lost, because the rider shifts position before settling back down again. And, of course, holding such an extreme position for a long time can cause physical damage. So for longer time trials a modicum of comfort or sustainability is important to the fit.

Crit/circuit/track racing

For an hour-long crit or circuit race, or even shorter bunch races on the track, comfort or sustainability are not massive considerations, but power production and, if you're intending to try and escape the bunch, aerodynamics are the priorities, so the pillars don't look too different to a time trial. In a bunch race scenario, though, there's an added consideration of bike feel and handling, and obviously you're not allowed to use tri-bar extensions!

Sportive

For a sportive rider – say you are taking on the Étape du Tour – the game changes completely. This is where goal-setting is really important. Unless you practise by riding for twice the duration of the event weekly, comfort has to be your number one aim. Finishing a hilly stage of the Tour is the goal for many people, but so many of them scupper themselves attempting it in a position that isn't built around allowing them to sit in the saddle for eight hours. Many bike manufacturers now produce models with 'endurance geometry' that are more suited to attaining this kind of position.

Gravel/adventure

Moving further along the comfort/sustainability spectrum, we have gravel and adventure riders. With huge and often multiple days in the saddle, and the additional load of luggage on the bike, power

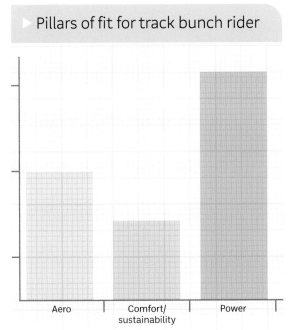

Pillars of fit for track bunch rider

Aero | Comfort/sustainability | Power

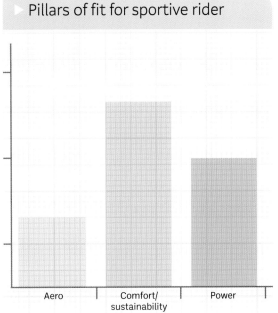

Pillars of fit for sportive rider

Aero | Comfort/sustainability | Power

production is still important, but comfort/sustainability is king. Interestingly, many gravel and adventure riders do fit tri-bars or similar extensions, but this isn't so much about getting aero, it's more about creating just another position to help share the load.

Commuter

At the polar end of the spectrum from a track pursuiter is a commuter, or someone who just has a bike to ride to the shops. There's no performance pressure or expectations on this type of cycling, so it's all about what feels good.

Comfort vs sustainability

When I was working with Team Sky and discussing the three pillars of fit with the support and coaching staff, I'd swap the word comfort for sustainability. The needs and demands of professional cycling often negate the notion of comfort. There's also a mindset that the riders are being paid too much to be comfortable if positions being merely tolerable means they win more!

Goal setting

In setting your goals and determining your optimal fit, be realistic; some of us are more adaptable than others, but all bikes have some level of adjustability. Adjust the bike yourself initially to take account of your level of adaptability, for example, how much you can bend your lower back to achieve a lower front-end position, or whether you can accept sitting on a narrow saddle for hours on end.

In setting out to examine your bike position, ask yourself the following questions:

What's your goal?

- ▶ Complete a sportive for the first time: prioritise comfort over power and aerodynamics.
- ▶ Go faster in a 25-mile time trial than ever before: prioritise aerodynamics and power over comfort.
- ▶ Ride and complete the Étape de Tour: prioritise comfort over aerodynamics and power.

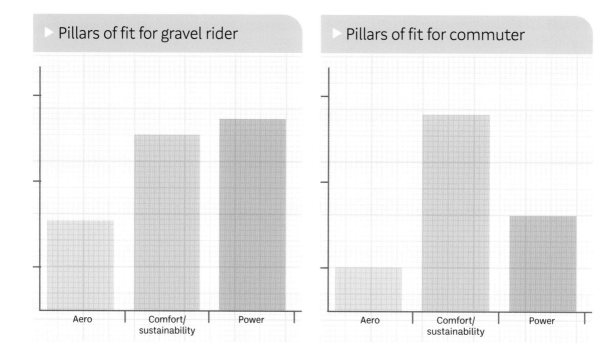

▶ Pillars of fit for gravel rider

Aero | Comfort/sustainability | Power

▶ Pillars of fit for commuter

Aero | Comfort/sustainability | Power

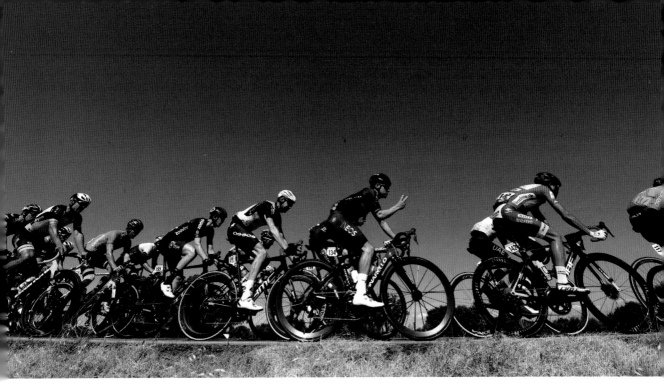

How much time do you have to devote to that goal?

▶ Very little: accept that you won't have time to adapt your body, so adjust your bike or reassess your goal.

▶ Lots: invest in bike fit and start to work on your limitations (for example, hamstring flexibility).

Evolution not revolution

All positions are evolved; no one immediately gets into an ideal position. Some involve a lot more work than others, but all are evolved. I was involved in collecting intelligence on injuries to cyclists as part of a massive audit into the area of injury by UK Sport. The most common causes of injury were sudden major changes in training volume and/or bike position. The body breaks down in pain or injury when it is asked to accept too much of a change without a sufficient period of time for adaptation. This is why I always evolve a position step by step. Even if it is fundamentally wrong to start with, if someone has been riding like that for a long time they are going to need time to adapt, even to a much better position.

An unnamed directeur sportif took a newly signed rider – who went on to win several Tour stages – and dropped his handlebars 3cm at the front end to make him more aerodynamic. He returned from the first team training ride in pain and with both hamstrings in spasm.

In many sports now – not just cycling – the interface between biology (human) and engineering (equipment) is where people are looking for gains in performance. For most of us, being realistic about our level of adaptability and letting the bike position reflect this will result in a safe, comfortable bike position.

If I look back on my notes of my time with British Cycling and specifically the saddle height of the men's Olympic track endurance squad tracked with age, a remarkable observation can be made. They all, slowly, evolved their saddle height upwards in small increments to an optimal height. This being the Holy Grail of power, it's an indirect measure of the adaptation they performed in order to be competitive.

Of course, not every position is attainable for every person: you have to be realistic. If you spend 38 hours a week sat at a desk and only manage two two-hour rides at the weekend, the competition for your body will be 'won' by the chair and desk. This will be exaggerated by any underlying medical history. Lower back pain and/or stiffness is a particularly common reason for people being unable to adopt a particular position. But don't despair: the best positions are evolved over time rather than being set in stone and forcing the body to adapt to them. If a sensible plan is made, most people can realise their goals on a bike with a position that works for them, it just might not involve them looking like a World Tour pro.

If someone comes to me with the goal of getting their saddle height higher to achieve a greater power output while time trialling and we discover the limiting factors are incredibly tight hamstrings and limited lumbar spine flexibility, we don't just give up. But neither do we ignore the problem and place them in a higher saddle height position. Instead we make a plan. Time spent riding in a slightly raised saddle position will allow the hamstrings to gradually adapt to lengthening a little more. If this is complemented with a progressive flexibility and stretching programme for the individual, over time most people can adapt to some extent to achieve their goal.

▶ Adaptation

The interaction between human and machine

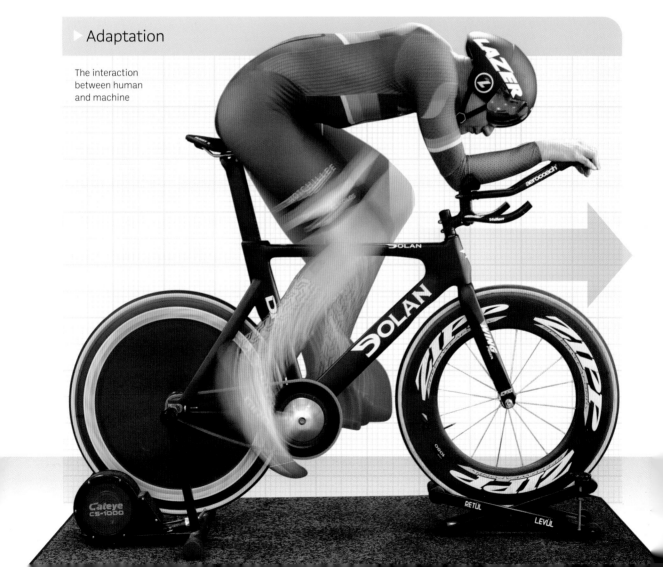

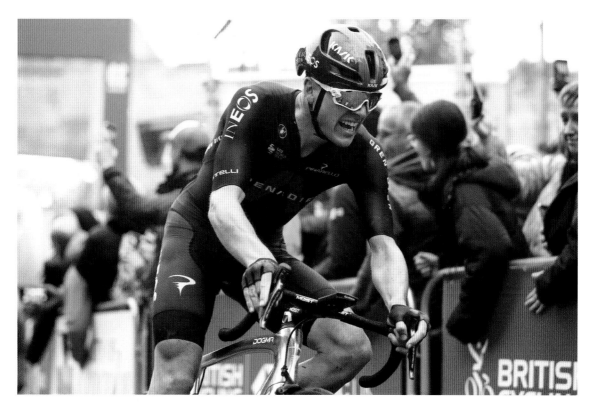

Micro-adjusters and macro-absorbers

I'm often asked how important optimising bike fit is. My most honest answer is: 'To some, very. To others, not so much.' I doubt you'll ever hear that from any commercial fitter, but it's my opinion and here's why.

In my first three years at Team Sky we did over 500 bike fits and data captures. This was with riders we knew well and followed up with constantly. That's quite a unique position to observe from. Alongside this, medical screenings are common in elite sports and provide another data stream. In examining all this data I started to notice a trend. I use something I call the spare bike index to help describe it. This refers to how long an individual can ride a bike position that isn't their own spot-on set-up before they feel pain or have to stop.

Ability to adapt is one of the most important things that separates us all in our ability to perform. Athletes all have to adapt to training, conditions, tactics – the list is endless. But why doesn't everyone do this to

the same degree? I noticed a trend: the people who micro-adjusted their position or were very sensitive to any changes in it generally scored as low adapters and were at increased risk of injury according to medical screenings.

The people who never adjusted their position, or were less susceptible to changes in it, scored as high adapters and were at decreased risk of injury. I termed these people macro-absorbers. They were able to absorb large changes or adapt to them without issues. In short: to the micro-adjusters bike position is very important and to macro-absorbers it's less important.

The annals of cycling record many a cyclist who constantly fiddled with their position: the most famous was Eddy Merckx, who constantly put his saddle up and down, carrying an Allen key in his pocket during races. In other words, he micro-adjusted. Many professional riders do this, probably to offload the muscles of the thigh before returning to position when they have recovered. But with others it is more a twitch – almost a superstition – searching for the optimum when it can't actually be reached. This fiddling acts as a psychological crutch: if I can get it perfect everything else will slot into place.

If someone changes something about the world they try to work with, be it desk set-up in the office or the set-up of their bike, a micro-adjuster will know about it straight away. World Tour pro and world track champion Ben Swift is one such rider. Ben will swear blind his saddle height is wrong when he simply has a new saddle that doesn't flatten down quite as much as the old one when he sits on it.

Ben's Spare Bike Index is six minutes 32 seconds. In other words, if Ben's team leader had a crash and Ben lent him his bike and had to ride someone else's spare one that's how long he would last before starting to feel pain and dysfunction.

Tour de France winner Geraint Thomas soaks up training stress like no one else and has ridden half a stage of the Tour de France on someone else's bike without even noticing. His spare bike index is three hours plus.

I know Ben and Geraint very well. The amount of time Ben spends off the bike on prehab and rehab to keep him optimal is truly amazing, whereas 'G' spends little or no time on such things. The two shapes below I think help to explain why. Ben's triangle, steep sided, has a very narrow pointed peak. This represents his absolute maximum ability to perform. Imagine a ball balanced on top of the peak: that's Bens cycling performance. The energy required to keep the ball from rolling down one side of the triangle is significant, because a slight movement will cause the ball to roll down one side, affecting either performance or injury avoidance.

G's adaptability is represented by a trapezoid with a wide, flat top, and the ball can roll a long way before his performance or injury status changes. A less-than-optimal bike position (a ball mover, so to speak) isn't as big a deal for him as it is for Ben.

If you recognise some of the traits of a micro-adjuster in yourself you'd be wise to pay attention to your interaction with the bike. It may well explain some of your past issues. However, there's no need to be neurotic and fall victim to the Eddy Merckx syndrome.

Geraint Thomas is a Macro-Absorber

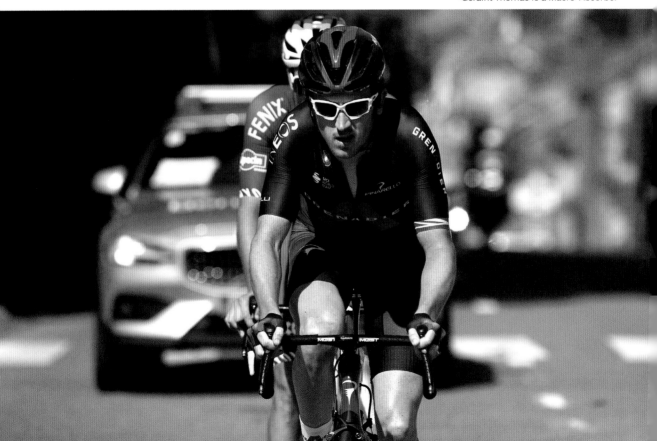

► The difference between micro-adjusters and macro-absorbers

PHYSIO SCORE ROBUSTNESS
VS FUNCTIONAL MOVEMENT
SCREENING

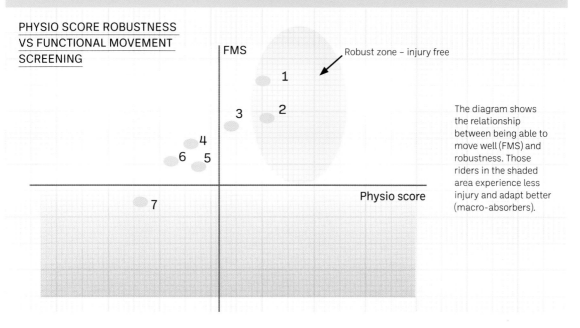

The diagram shows the relationship between being able to move well (FMS) and robustness. Those riders in the shaded area experience less injury and adapt better (macro-absorbers).

► Adaptability shapes

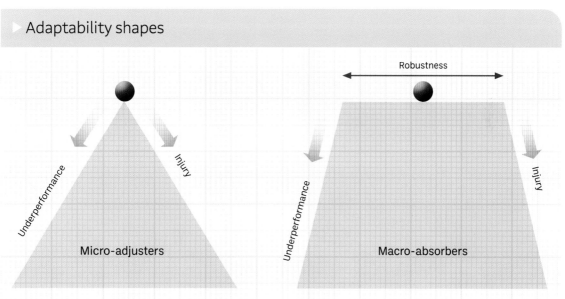

MICRO-ADJUSTERS VS MACRO-ABSORBERS

Note the narrow peak of the top level of the performance of a micro-adjuster. It takes very little energy to move the ball off the top – as in real life, it takes only small changes to inflict injury or lower performance. Compare this with the plateau of macro-absorbers and their ability to absorb changes.

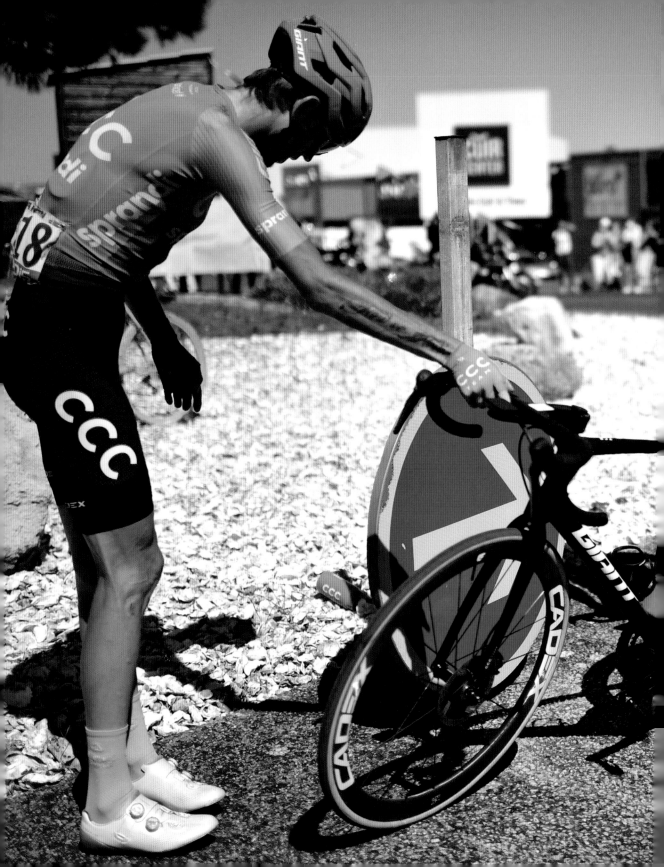

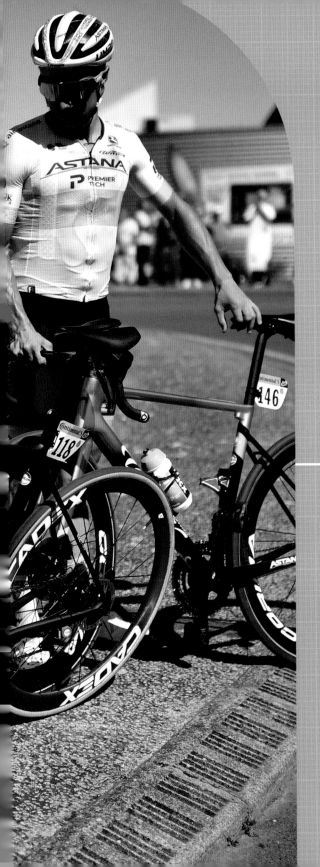

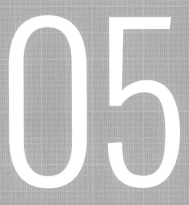

05

When problems occur

When problems occur

There is a distinct lack of injury-related research in cycling, partly due to the fact that you can't carry out cause-and-effect research into injuries, because it is unethical to set out to injure someone.

The waters are further muddied by the fact that elite and leisure cyclists tend to suffer from different complaints. A study by Clareson et al. (2010), a questionnaire given to 116 professional cyclists, revealed a trend similar to the one shown by the audit I conducted at British Cycling: the main injuries suffered by cyclists were knee, lower back and neck, in that order. Among the endurance cycling group these injuries rarely stopped a professional from racing or training. They did, however, require a lot of medical attention and it's by monitoring this that other studies have identified the level to which endurance cycling loads the body at certain points.

Foot/ankle

The importance of good fitting shoes can't be underestimated. The wrong shoes are going to impact negatively on your comfort, potentially your knee health and your power production. You don't generate any power below the knee, but you can lose plenty. For this reason, trying pairs on in a shop rather than just taking a punt online is always recommended. It's quite possible that you may require insoles or shims, so this has to be taken into account when fitting and choosing shoes too.

Feet vary in more than just the dimension of length or 'shoe size'. Accordingly, your shoe must fit your foot

▶ Different foot shapes

MAXIMAL VERSUS SUBMAXIMAL CYCLING: AN IMPORTANT DEFINITION

What most people are referring to when discussing cycling is submaximal cycling, cycling that relates to a power output and bike speed that is sustainable for a prolonged period of time. Maximal cycling refers to an all-out unpaced effort. It's important to define the two, as what holds true for one doesn't necessarily hold true for the other. For example, the relative importance and role of the hip flexors in submaximal cycling is negligible, but in maximal cycling it is crucial. Think about a track sprinter getting off the start line or launching his sprint attack.

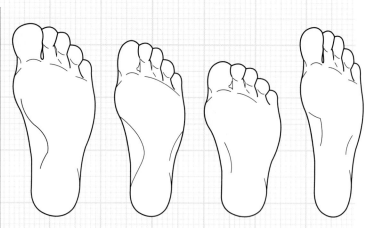

Feet vary in more than just the the dimension of length or 'shoe size'. Accordingly, your shoe must fit your foot shape as well as foot length.

shape as well as foot length.

Our feet and ankles are responsible for transferring the power generated in our legs to the pedals. Unlike running or walking there is no heel-strike or toe-off, and therefore no 'gait cycle' to speak of. Cyclists rarely suffer the multitude of aches, pains and injuries associated with running sports, largely due to the absence of the forces involved in repeatedly landing and loading the foot with multiples of body weight. However, problems of a different, if less severe, nature can and do arise.

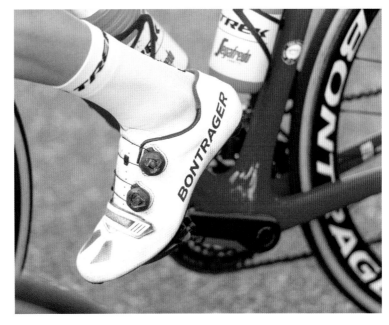

'Hot foot'

'Hot foot', numbness and tingling are complaints often reported by cyclists. The most common cause of these issues – and the first thing to check – is your footwear. As you cycle, your feet tend to swell slightly and the longer you cycle the more they swell. If your cycling shoe is too small or over-tightened the foot has nowhere to expand into. This squeezes the nerves and blood vessels, resulting in temporary numbness and tingling. You may have experienced the same 'dead' sensation when you have slept heavily on an arm or leg.

If you experience hot foot, check your cycling shoe size. Standing in the shoes unfastened should be comfortable, with no pressure on the toes.

▶ Different shoe shapes

Note the suble differences in the size of the toe box, height and wrap of the heel cup, and the heel-to-toe drop in height in these shoes from various manufacturers.

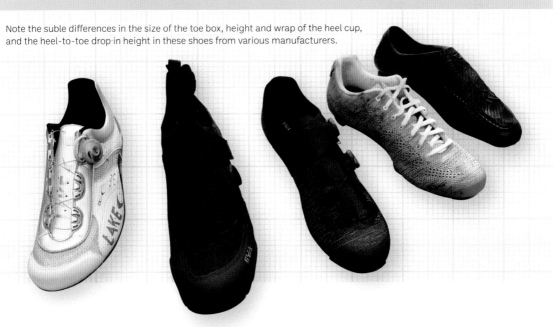

▶ Comparison of toe boxes

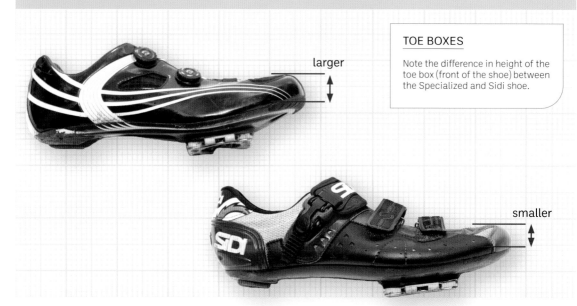

larger

smaller

TOE BOXES

Note the difference in height of the toe box (front of the shoe) between the Specialized and Sidi shoe.

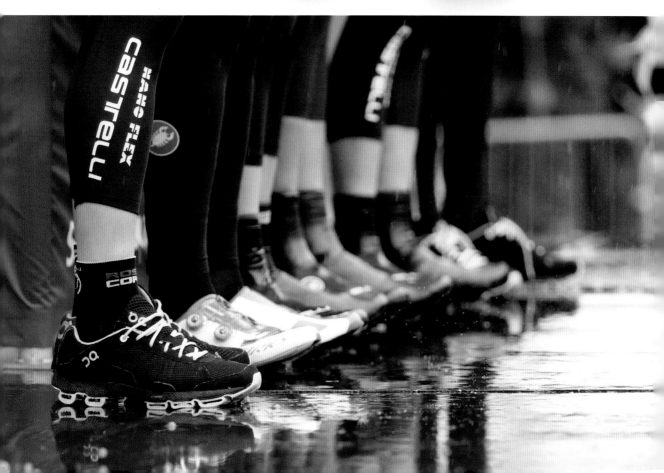

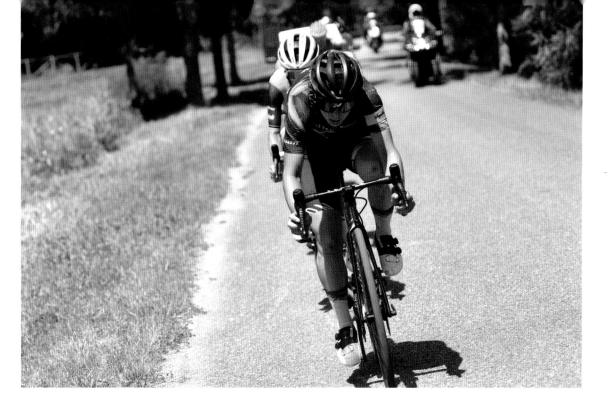

When fastened, they should still feel comfortable but when you lift your heel it should stay firmly in the shoe (i.e. the shoe should come up with the heel).

Try different ways and levels of fastening. Everyone's feet are different shapes, even though they are the same size. So one person may need a lot more tension/ fastening around the lower portion of the foot compared with the top end, and vice versa. Experiment with your fastening if you believe your shoe size to be correct. Sometimes it's not the size of the shoe that's the problem, but the shape. It's logical that differently shaped feet can be better accommodated by differently shaped shoes. See how differently shaped the shoes are in the photos.

The toe box – the available room in the front of the shoe for the toes – is roomy in a Specialized shoe but

▶ High arch and flat arch

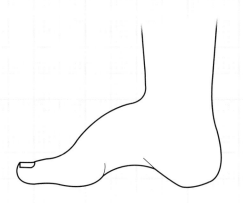 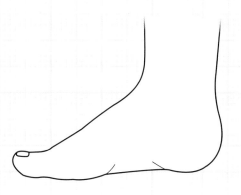

limited in a Sidi, which has a flatter, wider style.

More rarely, numbness and tingling can be caused by the nervous system being placed under undue stress or compression. Most commonly, this will be in cyclists who have a saddle height that's too high, forcing the leg to hyperextend at the knee – this can stretch a tight neural system and give the symptoms described. However, it is usually also associated with a line of posterior thigh pain.

Cramping

If you experience cramping of any sort always evaluate your fluid intake as this is the primary cause in most cases. However, cramping specific to the foot while cycling can be caused by wrong-sized shoes. Too small and the muscles of the foot cannot lengthen. Too large and the toes tend to curl constantly, seeking stability within the shoe.

Pain in the arch of the mid-foot often relates to the foot posture of the individual. Some people have a high arched foot posture, while others are very flat footed. The latter tend to over-pronate (flatten the arch of the foot) and, if not supported by the shape of the inside of the shoe or insole, this can cause problems. Some cycling shoes come with a range of insoles or orthotic devices that can help remedy this. Seeking the advice of a podiatrist is recommended if the problem isn't easily resolved.

Pain on the outside of the foot

Too tight a shoe will often cause pain around the fifth metatarsal head (the bony protruding joint of the pinky toe). I've seen an increase in riders experiencing this with the advent of carbon shoes in which the carbon sole wraps up and around the outside of the foot. The carbon is so unforgiving that the fit has to be spot-on to avoid any problems, but I've seen even custom-made versions thrown in the bin at great cost.

Another reason for pain on the outside of the foot is what some term 'waterfalling'. This is where the foot falls over the outside of the pedal with the shoe. It results from the cleat being positioned too far inward on the shoe, meaning there is too much unsupported pressure on the outside of the shoe. This normally occurs

▶ Stance-width correction to address waterfalling

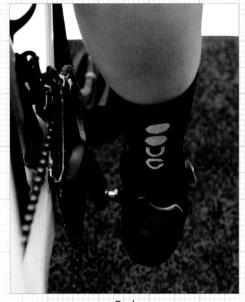

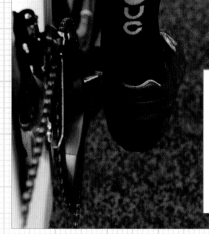

Here, with the cleat moved from the inside to the centre of the shoe, the foot no longer falls over the outside edge of the shoe.

Bad

Good

Carbon lip on outside of the foot

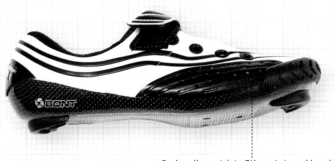

Carbon lip restricts 5th metatarsal head

in heavy and/or powerful riders – over time the shoe material breaks down and becomes soft, which allows the waterfalling (or overspill) action to occur. To solve the problem the underlying reason behind the inward cleat set-up must be addressed. This can happen in riders trying to get the foot away from the crank arm, because they are experiencing issues with their stance width –

duck-footed riders hitting the rear chainstays as their heels drop in, pedal systems with small Q factors (i.e. short spindle lengths) or riders with wider pelvises. Waterfalling is often easily addressed by increasing the rider's stance width (see pages 74–75) by using longer pedal spindles, or spacers.

Heel and Achilles tendon

Pain at the back of the heel or in the Achilles tendon can be really problematic for a cyclist. Footwear, pedalling technique and saddle height are the main causes.

The way a shoe cups your heel varies enormously. Too high and it can rub the Achilles and cause pain as the heel lifts in and out of the shoe. Too low and it will rub the heel bone. Some manufacturers are now adding directionally restrictive material to the heel cup to stop the heel lifting at all.

The way a shoe cups your heel can vary enormously

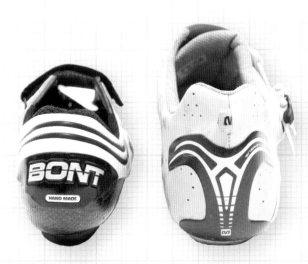

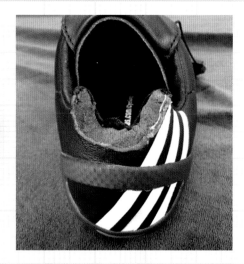

Note the difference in the heel cups. The material of the Mavic shoe on the right extends far higher and becomes narrower than the Bont shoe on the left. Riders with sensitive Achilles tendons may prefer less contact with their heel.

Many pros are sponsored by manufacturers to wear a brand of shoe. This can be quite lucrative, but sometimes the shoes don't work for the rider. Here is one World Champion's solution to a problematic heel cup they were contracted to wear!

▶ Heel-down pedalling

▶ Heel-to-toe drop

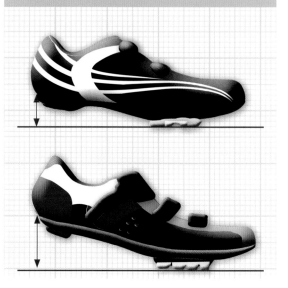

In a heel-down pedalling style, at bottom dead centre the knee is extended and the foot dorsiflexed (heel is down).

A shoe with less of a heel-to-toe drop results in a lower heel position.

▶ The effects of saddle height

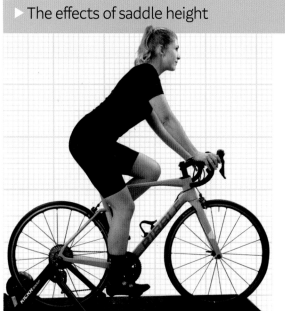

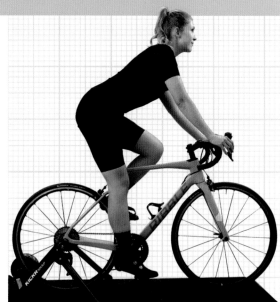

SADDLE TOO LOW CAUSING HEEL-DOWN PEDALLING

Note how the rider has absorbed the low saddle height by dorsiflexing the foot more and thus preserving a good knee angle.

SADDLE TOO HIGH CAUSING OVERREACH

Again note how the body attempts to absorb the high saddle at the ankle rather then the knee by plantarflexing (toes down) the foot.

Your footwear should also suit your pedalling style. If you pedal with your heels down, a change to a shoe that has less of a heel-to-toe drop will result in an even lower heel position at BDC.

Heel and Achilles pain can also be caused by a saddle that is the wrong height. Too low a saddle can force a very heel-down pedalling style onto the rider, while a high saddle will make a rider overreach constantly with the foot.

Sustained hill climbing can cause Achilles issues unless you are used to it. On long climbs we tend to adopt a rearward-seated, leg-extended, heel-down pedalling style to conserve energy and this places more stress on the Achilles tendon. The Great Britain Olympic sprint cycling squad, who rarely cycle for longer than 90 minutes at a time, experienced these issues when they went for their annual training at the endurance camp in Majorca and found themselves out for longer and hillier rides than they were used to.

Achilles issues can linger even after the initial cause has been addressed. A simple solution that often works is to move your cleats backwards. This reduces the load on the tendon by shortening the lever arm of the foot to the pedal.

Foot/cleat canting

As one of the major contact points between bike and human, the foot/pedal interface and its set-up are very important. There has been a substantial expansion in the products available to allow for adjustment of this and it's easy to see why. The repetitive nature of cycling means that if this set-up is off, for example due to

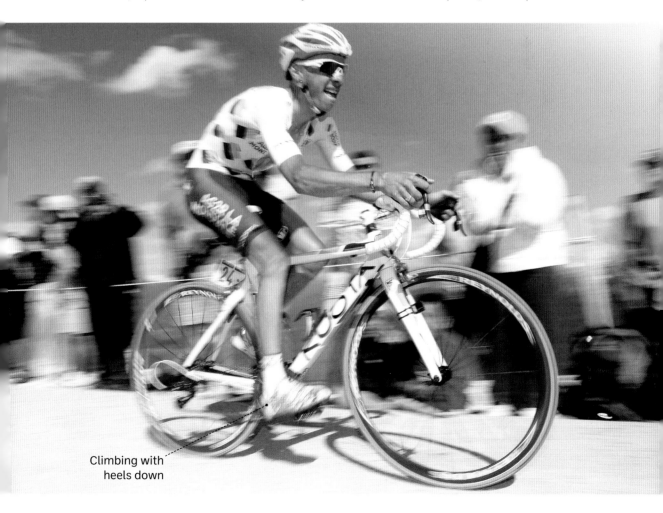

Climbing with heels down

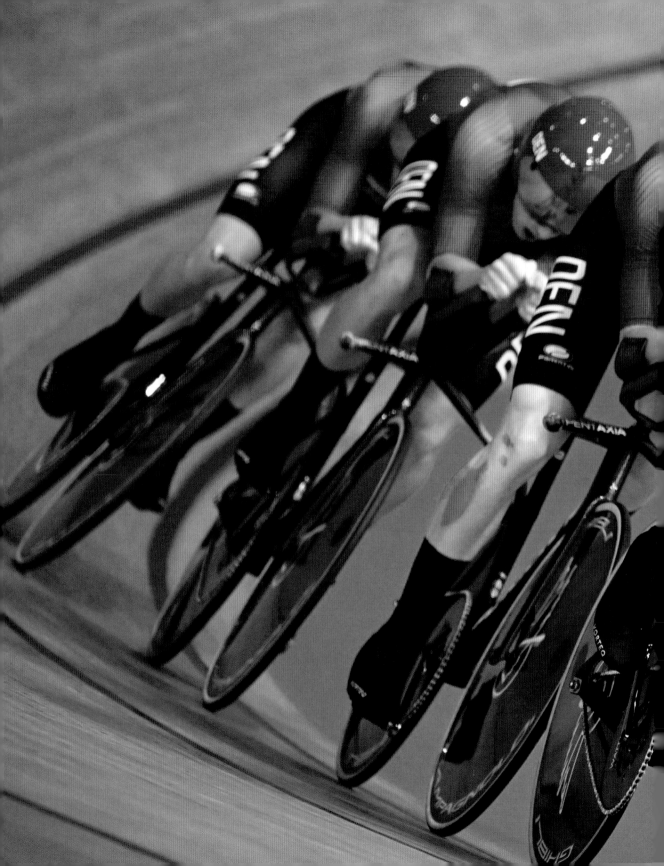

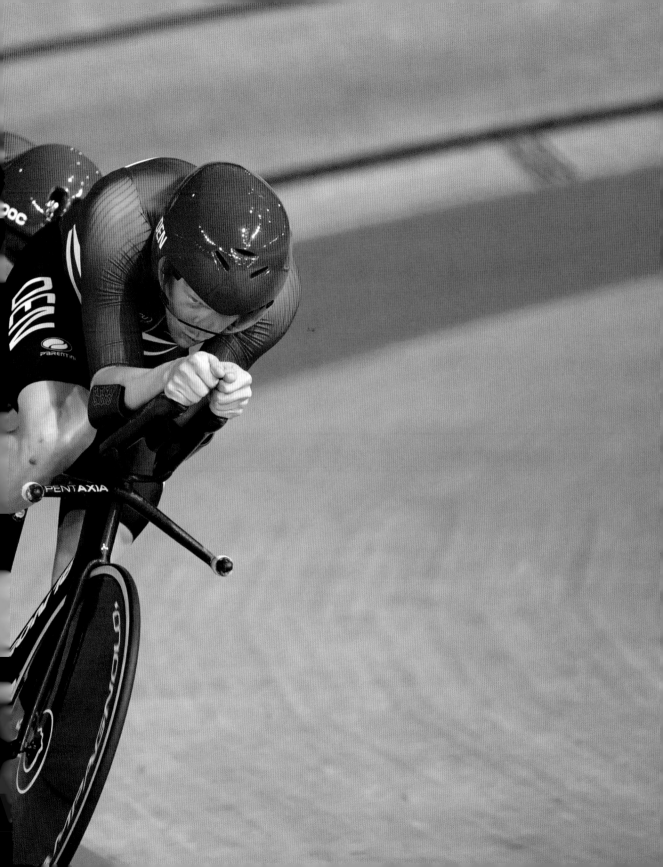

abnormal foot biomechanics, you may be predisposed to overuse injuries at the ankle, knee or hip – the kinetic chain. This chain is influenced by the forces developed at the foot, hence the importance of this contact point in bike set-up. However, the assessment and prescription of corrective interventions to the kinetic chain is controversial due to its medical nature and there is potential for harm if done poorly.

FOOT BIOMECHANICS

As far as I'm concerned, the foot is by far the most amazing structure in the body. When we walk it alternates within milliseconds between being a soft and supple structure that can adapt to whatever surface it encounters to a rigid lever propelling us forward. Between these two distinct functions the human foot goes through a mechanism of pronation and supination.

The podiatrist at British Cycling and I developed a simple way of looking at an abnormal foot so we could work together when trying to solve problems. 'Abnormal' generally means anything that is either too rigid or too flexible. The normal foot naturally pronates

a modest amount upon bearing weight. An excessively flexible foot pronates too much and is visible as a flat arch. An excessively rigid foot does not pronate much at all on weight bearing and maintains a visibly high – or supinated – arch. Due to the complex nature of the foot, interventions in this area have been left to the medical community and specialists. In cycling, however, the foot only has to act as a rigid lever, and there is no heel strike, only toe-off. This makes the role of supporting the cycling foot somewhat easier, because it does not have to balance the conflicting demands of firm and soft that walking requires.

There are two basic interventions to correct feet in cycling – internal orthotics or external shims. Internal orthotics are sculpted insoles and can be off the shelf or custom made. External shims work by being placed between the cleat and the shoe to 'cant' the entire shoe either inwards (valgus) or outwards (varus). The shimming boom started from the realisation that you could correct foot mechanics in cycling at the forefoot and support its function as a rigid lever. Indeed, many peddled the idea that traditional mid-rear foot

▶ Foot issues

SOURCE	CAUSE	SOLUTION
Foot pain/numbness	Cycling shoes too tight	Loosen straps – feet swell when cycling
		Change shoe size
		Remove insole or change size to accommodate
	Ball of foot pain	Move cleat – follow guidelines
	Waterfalling – pain on outside of foot	Move cleat in to move foot out – consider longer spindles
Foot cramping	Shoes too small	Change size
	Shoes too big (toes overwork to gain stability)	Change size
Achilles pain	Saddle too high	Reduce height – stop foot overreaching
	Saddle too low	Increase height – stop heel-down pedalling style
	Sustained hill climbing	Avoid until settled or move cleat backwards
	Cleat position too far forward	Move cleat backwards to lessen load on Achilles

correction was useless as the forefoot was where the foot made contact with the pedal.

Canting the whole shoe has a much more powerful effect than simply supporting someone's arch within it. It affects the entire kinetic chain through the limb: hip, knee and ankle. Many authorities have promoted the kinetic chain effect of shimming to correct, for example, frontal knee tracking so the knee becomes more vertically linear. However, there is little evidence to support this and some strong evidence that it may do more harm than good (Ruby et al. 1992).

There is also a widely used, but highly inflated, quote in cycling that 80 per cent of the population have forefoot varus, and should therefore have their feet shimmed with varus wedges to improve the connection with the pedal and eliminate unwanted excessive pronation. In my experience, this simply is not true, which brings us to the crux of the problem. Assessing forefoot varus and valgus and foot biomechanics in general is very difficult and may explain the over-reporting of forefoot varus in the cycling population.

In my opinion, we should not try to cant or wedge riders' shoes unless there is a well-thought-out and medically assessed reason to do so (such as an overuse injury or abnormal biomechanics), or the rider already uses a canted orthotic in everyday life.

The simple rule for me is this: look to support your foot's natural weighted alignment, allowing your foot to sit how it wants to sit. Do not attempt to correct foot mechanics beyond your normal mechanical structure unless aided by an appropriately qualified individual.

Knee

The knee is the most commonly injured or painful joint in cyclists. There are a great many factors behind the various issues that can affect the knee. This is partly because the knee joint is the unsupported joint (i.e. it is not in contact with the bike), which helps transfer the power generated from the pelvis and upper leg to the foot/ankle and ultimately the pedal. The way the contact points at the pelvis (saddle) and foot (pedal)

Pronation and supination

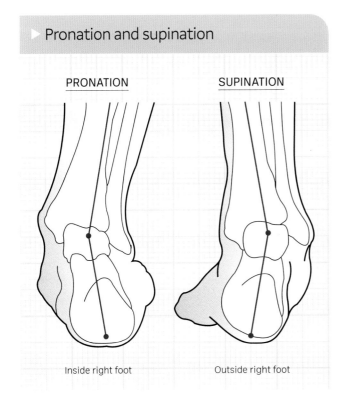

PRONATION   SUPINATION

Inside right foot   Outside right foot

Forefoot varus and valgus

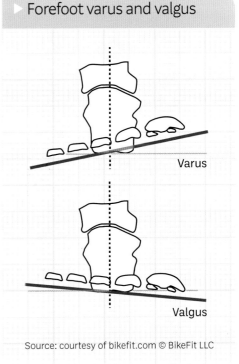

Varus

Valgus

Source: courtesy of bikefit.com © BikeFit LLC

are set up affects the knee. As you can imagine, there are a very large number of combinations of variables that can lead to the same issues. A great many cycling knee injuries occur due to an inappropriate load being placed on the joint in a repetitive manner. When you are running and fall off a curb your ankle may compensate for the action and the very next step will use a different loading pattern. In cycling, if you lock your feet into the foot/pedal interface incorrectly, in the next hour any abnormal load on a particular tissue inside your knee could be repeated several thousand times. Cycling knee injuries are largely caused by non-optimal ergonomics (i.e. bad bike fit) or large changes in training load.

The literature to date has often left this complicated area to either an oversimplified table of symptoms and causes or in-depth biomechanical descriptions which leave the rider to figure out what has caused their problem on their own. Also, a number of less-than-helpful myths exist regarding how the knee tracks or should track (see page 110).

In spite of all this it is worth being clear here that for people with knee injuries cycling is actually a very safe form of exercise for rehabilitation and future sport. Many a rehab specialist will use cycling as the first form of cardiovascular exercise for a patient recovering from a knee injury, due to its partial weight-bearing nature and relatively safe 2D plane of movement.

I hope to explain here how you can recognise your problem, understand why it is happening and come up with a solution. To make this as clear as possible we need to talk briefly about the way we will be looking at the knee. We will use the side view (sagittal plane) to explain saddle height, saddle fore/aft and pedal fore/aft.

Cyclists' knee problems can most often be addressed by examining the loading pattern and modifying the bike set-up or training load, combined with some remedial work off the bike. Hence we will concentrate on the reasons for knee injury, not the definitions of individual complaints. It's worth mentioning that almost all of the bike fitting

▶ Planes of view

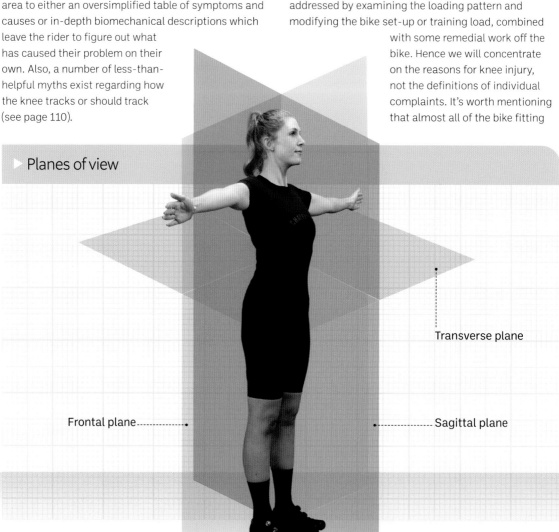

Transverse plane

Frontal plane

Sagittal plane

► Knee issues

SOURCE	CAUSE	SOLUTION
Front (anterior) pain	Saddle too low	Raise saddle to optimal knee angle for riding style
	Saddle too far forward	Move backwards
	Cranks too long	Shorten
	Cleats too far forward	Move rearwards
Inside (medial) pain	Saddle too low	Raise saddle to optimal knee angle for riding style
	Saddle too high	Lower saddle to optimal knee angle for riding style
	Cleat position	Should reflect walking style – heels in walking, allow heels to drop in on pedals
	Excessive float	Dial float off or change to a cleat with less float, check for worn cleats, pedals
	Stance width too wide (feet too far apart)	Reduce stance width – move cleats in and/or change spindle length to pedal
Outside (lateral) pain	Saddle too high	Lower saddle to optimal knee angle for riding style
	Saddle too low	Raise saddle to optimal knee angle for riding style
	Cleat positioning	Should reflect walking style – heels-in walking, allow heels to drop in on pedals
	Excessive float	Dial float off or change to a cleat with less float, check for worn cleats, pedals
	Stance width too narrow (feet too close together)	Increase stance width – move cleats out and/or change spindle length of pedal
Back (posterior) pain	Saddle too high	Lower saddle to optimal knee angle for riding style
	Saddle too far back	Move forward
	Reach too far	Relax/shorten reach to allow pelvis to rotate back – loosening hamstrings
	Saddle shape	Can block pelvic rotation – change to allow

NB: Shortening cranks can help to facilitate many of these changes and hence resolve issues.

interventions that can have an impact on knee health can be facilitated by switching to shorter cranks.

You will hear people describe patella tendonitis, patella maltracking, anterior knee pain and plica as the given diagnosis of their knee pain on the bike. It's my experience that unless the medical practitioner examining you has a working knowledge of cycling you will most probably end up with a diagnosis related to off-the-bike activity. This is fine if it's correct, but if the

injury is caused by being on the bike they are unlikely to properly address the cause.

A fine example is apparent plical problems. These are the cause of more debate than any other tissue in the cyclist's knee. Plicae are small folds around the joint and some say they are a pointless bit of kit left over from babyhood. Surgeons disagree over their relative importance, but the problem is that they often appear on MRI scans as inflamed and are usually (to my mind) wrongly identified as the cause of pain. Most surgical cases are complicated and long, and it can be hard to say whether a procedure worked or whether merely enforcing a rehabilitation programme and rest period improved the knee anyway. I would exhaust all biomechanical interventions before reverting to plica removal or cortisone injection.

For this reason, if you want an accurate diagnosis of a knee injury caused by cycling alone, try your best to locate a cycling-knowledgeable physio or doctor, or at least someone with an open mind.

Knee – side, or sagittal view

On page 42, the ideal knee joint angles for setting saddle height were described. These figures aren't just plucked out of the air. A knee extension angle of 30-35 degrees and knee flexion of 110 degrees at BDC and TDC respectively are recommended with good cause, as angles higher or lower than this can lead to problems.

Saddle height

Riding a saddle that is too high often leads to problems and pain at the back and outside of the knee. The hamstring muscles have to reach further than is comfortable – especially if they are already inflexible – and start to complain, often at the point where they attach to the back of the knee. The iliotibial band (ITB), the large sinuous band of muscle interwoven with fascia (flat tendon) that runs from the outside of the hip to outside of the knee, is also forced to extend beyond its functional length and this manifests itself as pain at the outside of the knee or the kneecap as it starts to pull sideways.

A high saddle can also cause calf pain, as the foot and ankle point down to reach the pedal at the bottom of the pedal stroke.

If you suspect your saddle height is too high, try employing the methods detailed on pages 42–48 to set it optimally. Alternatively, try lowering it slightly (0.5cm can make all the difference) and seeing if your symptoms improve.

Golden rule: change only one thing at a time when

▶ Knee position in the sagittal view

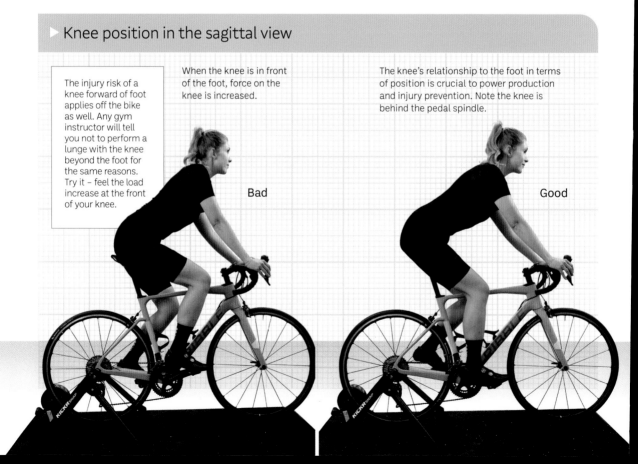

The injury risk of a knee forward of foot applies off the bike as well. Any gym instructor will tell you not to perform a lunge with the knee beyond the foot for the same reasons. Try it – feel the load increase at the front of your knee.

When the knee is in front of the foot, force on the knee is increased.

Bad

The knee's relationship to the foot in terms of position is crucial to power production and injury prevention. Note the knee is behind the pedal spindle.

Good

trying this, otherwise you will not know which change is working for you!

Riding a saddle height that is too low tends to cause pain at the front of the knee, around the kneecap. This is because of the increased compressive forces on the kneecap as the leg comes over the top of the pedal stroke and then pushes down.

Saddle fore/aft positioning can be seen as a component of saddle height, and motion analysis systems will calculate it as part of a function of height and setback, but it has its own relevance. If the position of the saddle is too far back, the saddle height is effectively increased, and riders often experience hamstring strain and/or pain at the back of the knee.

If the saddle is too far forward, pain at the front of the knee becomes the issue, as the knee comes in front of the foot. The more the knee joint comes in front of the foot in the pedalling cycle, the more compressive forces end up acting on the kneecap. In very simple terms, the kneecap is squashed against the front of the thigh bone. These compressive forces can cause anterior or front knee pain.

The set-up of the cleats on the shoe can affect the knee. If the cleat is too far forward the knee will also end up too far forward in relation to the foot and this can cause pain at the front of the knee.

Cleats positioned too far back (towards the arch of the foot) reduce the chance of the knee being forward of the foot, but also increase the distance the foot must travel. Again, if saddle height isn't optimal hamstrings can overstretch as they have to try and extend to reach the pedal position.

Coronal, or frontal view

Next time you are watching the Tour de France or any professional race, take a minute to examine the way the riders at the front of the race are moving.

The knee movement you see is often described as the knee 'tracking' relative to the hip and foot. I can guarantee that you will see many different tracking patterns. Some riders will have their knees out, some will have their knees in, and in some cases the knees do different things. These riders are competing in the top bike races in the world and yet many so-called bike-

▶ Knee tracking

As the rider pedals, the knees move in and out, towards and away from the top tube to varying degrees in different people.

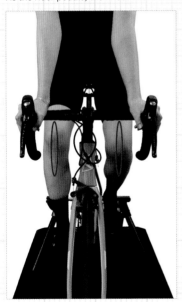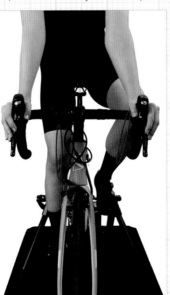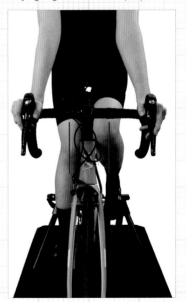

fitting experts would seek to fundamentally change the way their knee tracks in the frontal plane. This is because there are some commonly held – but to my mind misguided – beliefs regarding knee tracking.

The first of these preconceptions is that the hip, knee and foot should be aligned in a vertical plane while riding. The justification for this is that it is most effective for power production and transfer of that power to the pedal. From a purely mechanical angle one can see how movement of the knee away from the most direct path between the sources of power (the hip and knee) to the place of power transfer (the foot and ankle) can be considered wasteful in term of energy. However, studies conducted on this are limited and inconclusive at best, and in my view there is no strong evidence that deviating from the most direct path is harmful. In fact, the opposite may be true and in trying to align them we may cause harm.

A problem-solving approach

It's important when considering pain and dysfunction related to cycling to not only look at your equipment and set-up for the causes.

There can be a myriad of reasons for a pain or injury. It can be hard to fathom out what is going on, as often one thing can lead to another. Before long you find yourself chasing a problem that began as a mere niggle, but ends up as a serious threat to your cycling.

It's not the just the rank-and-file weekend amateurs either. I've helped world champions and Tour de France stage winners overcome relatively simple issues that have gone on for far too long, because the people helping them – physios, doctors and scientists – failed to see the wood for the trees. And not for want of trying; cycling is a unique sport with a unique injury profile.

Here's my simple guide to what we medical folk call differential diagnosis – or working out what's going on

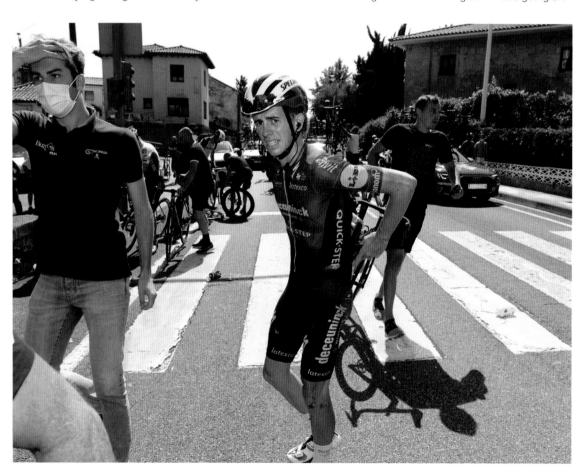

AEIOU: it's all in the vowels

Let's take one problem and work out what could be the reason for it happening.

A male cyclist has pain in his right knee. Using AEIOU we can work out why:

▶ A FOR ACTIVITY

Ask yourself if you've changed anything recently in the make-up of your training – the root cause might be large or abrupt changes in load, volume or terrain with possibly not enough time to adapt. Common reasons for knee pain are increased hill training, large amounts of big-gear riding, or simply a huge and dramatic increase in training volume.

Examine what you have been doing and if changes correlate with injury or pain issues, investigate further.

▶ E FOR EQUIPMENT

Ask yourself if anything has changed recently: shoes, cleats that may be new or worn, cleat position, pedal type, bike set-up, etc. There is much more detail on this elsewhere in the book. Changes in activity and equipment account for 75 per cent of all cycling injuries at British Cycling.

▶ I FOR INTRINSIC

Or 'you'! Intrinsic issues are those related to you and your body make-up. A difference in length between right and left leg can lead to knee pain, as can a twisted pelvis or a torn muscle healing with scar tissue in the thigh. Know your body; understand its unique set-up.

▶ O FOR OTHER

This is the category where we can place all those weird and wonderful reasons that actually make a lot of sense. A long-haul flight results in your knee not moving for eight hours and subsequently being stiff and painful. You've been ill for a week laid up in bed – unable to stretch or function – everything tightens and the right knee bears the brunt of this on your return to training and becomes sore.

An insect bite becomes badly infected and the subsequent swelling causes your kneecap to move irregularly, resulting in pain.

▶ U FOR UNKNOWN

Sometimes a pain or injury has a cause or reason that is not immediately obvious. The human body is an amazingly complicated structure and it continually defies complete knowledge of its working. But don't fear. If the cause is unknown you can often treat it by addressing what is known. Let's say you have knee pain. Optimise your position with the advice within these pages to accommodate that pain. Your position may not have been the cause of the issue, but by changing it to a knee-safe one you can help the issue resolve.

I honestly believe that by applying this rationale you can often work out 80 per cent of problems yourself. The preceding chapters help us work out the finer details of when the E for equipment and its set-up are responsible for the problem.

So our man with right knee pain?

He looks at his training and discovers he's in a pretty stable period and nothing much has changed – no A. Intrinsically he knows he has a leg-length difference, but this has been accounted for – no I. However, he hasn't replaced his cleats in some time and on examination the right cleat is completely loose. This could be the reason for his knee pain as the right leg would have been toggling around on the pedal, increasing the right workload to control the forces applied during pedalling. So E is the reason.

Preferred movement pathway

If you ask a random sample of people to do a task, whether it's pedalling or jumping up onto a box, there will be a huge variation in how that task is accomplished. This is simply because we all have our preferred movement patterns. Some might look more elegant or efficient than others, but none are wrong or need to be corrected unless they're causing pain, discomfort, injury or a drastic loss of power.

A great example of this is probably one of the greatest runners of all time, Michael Johnson. His running style was lambasted for not conforming to the style that was universally accepted as right. He was constantly told he would not make it in track and field, and coaches tried to change him, but he remained true to himself. I personally know of a UK Olympic long jumper who was successful with an unconventional run-up. The experts in the team thought he would jump even better if he changed his style to match the conventional run-up. His performance declined sharply. He returned to his old style and was successful again. It goes to show that if something looks odd, but works, it doesn't always hold that changing it will result in an even better performance. It may look odd, but it may be the only way the individual can achieve optimum performance.

▶ Forefoot varus

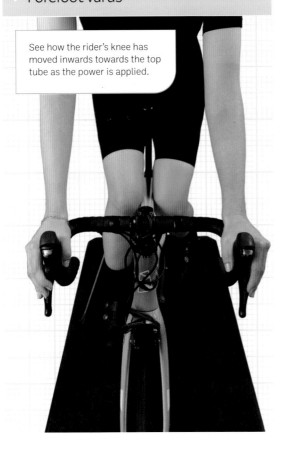

See how the rider's knee has moved inwards towards the top tube as the power is applied.

▶ A wedge and a shim

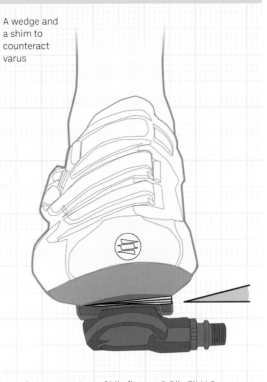

A wedge and a shim to counteract varus

Source: courtesy of bikefit.com © BikeFit LLC

by elimination and deduction, my dear Watson.

You will become aware of your knee tracking style as you cycle more and for longer; and I would not try changing any rider's frontal knee tracking unless they had an overuse pain or injury. Even then I would look for layers of evidence supporting the case that correcting the tracking would be beneficial before intervening. This is because a person's frontal knee tracking is often simply a reflection of their own unique biomechanics, injury history and abilities on a bike. Unfortunately, this goes against a whole industry that has sprung up around knee alignment theory, offering various interventions, the most common of which are wedges or shims. These are important and powerful interventions, and because they are exactly that – powerful – they need to be applied with sound reasoning (sometimes clinical).

Different knee tracking

There are different types of knee tracking, with different causes, and these differences are not necessarily problematic. Nevertheless, issues related to knee tracking do occur and we should cover the main culprits.

KNEES IN

A knees-in style of pedalling has been attributed to foot posture and mechanics. As the knee comes over top dead centre and power starts to be applied to the pedal through the ball of the foot, the action of the foot determines where the knee tracks. If the rider has forefoot varus (big toe is higher than little toe) it is argued that the foot over-pronates (i.e. the arch flattens) causing the knee to move towards the bike as it extends further. This is due to the tibia rotating on the femur

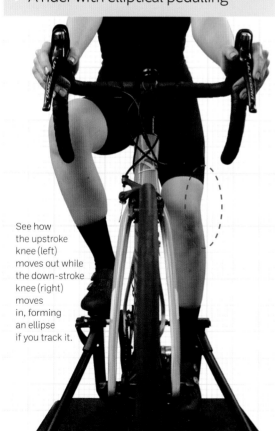

A rider with elliptical pedalling

See how the upstroke knee (left) moves out while the down-stroke knee (right) moves in, forming an ellipse if you track it.

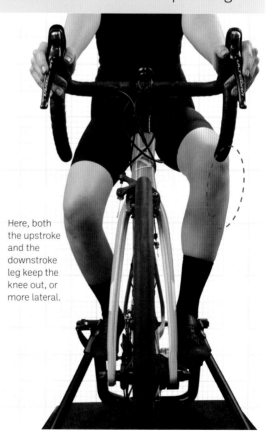

A rider with knees-out pedalling

Here, both the upstroke and the downstroke leg keep the knee out, or more lateral.

as the leg extends early to compensate for the foot reaching the end of its adjustability.

By correcting the forefoot varus using a varus wedge or shim under the cleat, this action, along with the deviation of the knee towards the centre of the bike, can be limited. Proponents of wedging quote that 80 per cent of the population have forefoot varus and therefore for better power production and alignment most riders should use varus wedging.

This figure has been vastly overestimated according to many foot specialists, who say true forefoot varus is rare. The disparity may well arise from bike fit specialists assessing the foot incorrectly, because it's quite a skill to establish the neutral position of the foot in order to measure for forefoot varus.

If you do have a knees-in riding style and are experiencing knee pain or problems, my advice is to look for reasons off the bike first. For example, do you wear corrective insoles or orthotics off the bike for an already identified foot mechanical or posture issue? If so, have you transferred these to your cycling shoes? If not, do so and see if it makes a difference.

If you haven't had your foot posture assessed, but are worried about it, seek medical advice from a registered podiatrist.

KNEES IN AND OUT

Some riders pedal in an elliptical fashion, with the knee moving inwards towards the bike on the downstroke and then away from the bike on the returning upstroke. This is very common and is more than likely down to riders externally rotating their hips after the pressure of the downstroke in order to unload the joint and return it to TDC to start the next pedal cycle. Some argue this

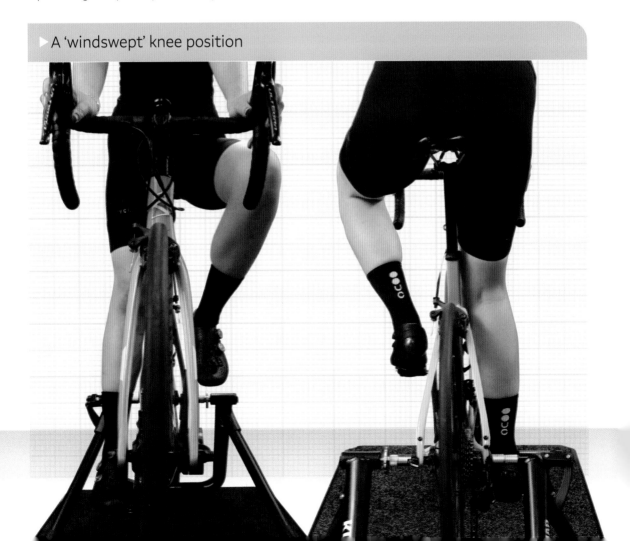

▶ A 'windswept' knee position

enables the hip flexors to work more effectively – but noting the work of many, such as Martin and Barrat (2009) (see the hip section on page 115), which has proved the negligible contribution of the hip flexors in the overall power profile of pedalling, this seems less important.

KNEES OUT

I often see a bow-kneed or knees-out style of pedalling in the city I commute through. The most common cause is someone riding a bike that is much too small for them, or with a very low saddle height, often because they have jumped on a bike for the first time or borrowed someone else's. I don't see this style of knee tracking very often at the top end of cycling, and if the bike and saddle height

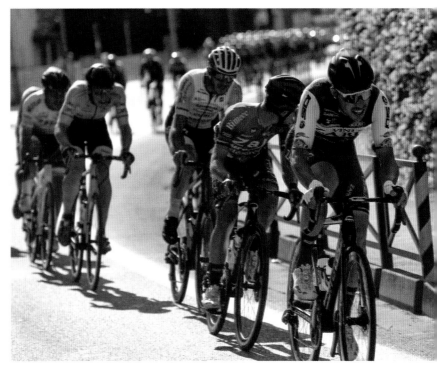

are optimal I would say it is a reflection of the rider's weight, hip and knee issues. Obese riders must take their knees out to the side to avoid their thighs coming into contact with their stomach. Riders with hip pain will naturally rotate their hips as much as possible to unload and therefore decrease the strain placed on the hip joint.

Riders with this style who are just starting out tend to see it normalise as they pedal more and lose weight. If it persists, increasing the stance width offers the best way to improve things. Just as varus wedges (see pages 129–131) are prescribed to correct knees coming in, valgus wedges can help a rider who pedals with knees out. However, forefoot valgus affects less than 10 per cent of people and caution should be used inserting wedges for the wrong reason as they can cause pain. In short, the best solution is probably either losing weight or getting a bigger bike!

KNEES IN ONE SIDE AND OUT THE OTHER, OR 'WINDSWEPT'

This style of frontal knee tracking is often associated with asymmetry – specifically a difference (either actual or functional – see page 129) in leg length –

or spinal issues resulting in a twisted pelvis. Addressing this style of pedalling, if it is causing problems, needs assessment and appropriate management by someone who is qualified to join up the rider's body limitations with the bike fit, a doctor or physio working in cycling. See pages 129–131 for information on anatomical differences and asymmetry.

OTHER PAINS

The amount of float in a cleat/pedal system can lead to issues at the knee. Cleats that have begun to wear out can cause excessive float, known as 'toggling', and side-to-side rocking. In trying to control the excess movement the knee can develop pain. Changing the type of float one uses can also cause issues.

Muscle imbalances

All of the above imbalances can lead to knee pain, and the list of possible knee injuries is huge, but there are some that crop up much more often than others.

RECTUS FEMORIS TIGHTNESS

This muscle is the one quad muscle to cross both the hip and knee joint (it's what we physios call a 'bilateral

Foam roller – the worst pain ever?

All of the riders at British Cycling and Team Sky were issued with foam rollers and I strongly recommend riders who come to see me for a bike fit to get one, too. A foam roller is a hard foam cylinder about 15cm in diameter. It is rolled over the muscle to ease pain and is a fantastic tool for releasing tight myofascial units around the body (i.e. where the muscles and fasciae connect). The ITB is a great example of a myofascial unit that can become too tight and dysfunctional. This often happens because of its role in controlling the knee throughout the repetitive nature of cycling. Anyone who has committed to a lot of regular cycling would benefit from using a foam roller to avoid picking up a knee niggle. Why wait for it to happen? If you have a knee issue and you or your therapist suspect the ITB is involved, foam rolling it can help remedy the issue.

Start by rolling slowly up and down on your side on top of the roller, keeping your feet off the floor and trying to put your entire body weight through your leg into the roller. Three sets of 10 rolls every day is a good effort. It will be very painful to begin with and can even bruise you, but do it every day for two weeks and, trust me, the pain goes away completely! I'd recommend all riders to maintain the functional length of the ITB by foam rolling just three times a week. For more detail on foam rollers, see below.

▶ Using a foam roller

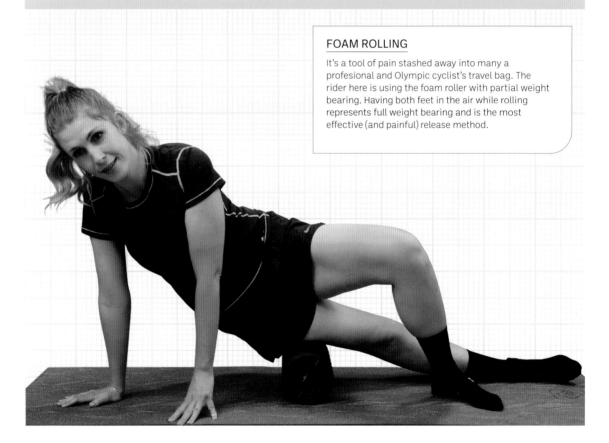

FOAM ROLLING

It's a tool of pain stashed away into many a profesional and Olympic cyclist's travel bag. The rider here is using the foam roller with partial weight bearing. Having both feet in the air while rolling represents full weight bearing and is the most effective (and painful) release method.

joint muscle'). In doing so, it can have two roles: extending the knee or flexing the hip. This quality gives it the ability to be used as a controlling or dampening muscle on the sheer power of the quadriceps muscles in the thigh. Unfortunately, it also means it's the first and most likely thigh muscle to become tight, restricting the smooth passage of the patella and therefore creating knee pain. Addressing this imbalance (see page 171) will very often be the key factor in relieving a cyclist's knee pain.

ILIOTIBIAL BAND TIGHTNESS OR DYSFUNCTION

Much debate exists to the exact role and nature of the ITB. Some argue it is a passive tendon-like structure, others that it is an active muscle in its own right. I believe it probably has elements of both. What I do know for certain is that ITB tightness provoked by an inappropriate Q angle (see page 75) due to positional errors will cause knee pain, and the way to relieve that is to address the cause – position, cleat set-up or stance width – and remove the tightness by using a foam roller.

Hips

Hip flexors

The hip flexors' importance in cycling has long been poorly interpreted. Many authors and experts have suggested these muscles are responsible for pulling up on the pedal on the upstroke and so the lack of power often seen on an upstroke's power profile is due to muscular inefficiency. Coaches have seized upon this as a reason to train with pedal coaching (pedalling in circles, for example). Innovative equipment has been developed, notably power cranks, which the rider has to pull up as they disengage and fall to BDC. However, with the work of Martin and Barrat (2009) and others it is clear now that this lack of power on the upstroke is due to non-muscular forces (rather than inefficiency) and that consciously trying to pull up more, or pedalling in circles, actually makes you more inefficient.

In fact, apart from helping to give maximum power from a standing start, the hip flexors make very little contribution to sustained pedal power. The contribution

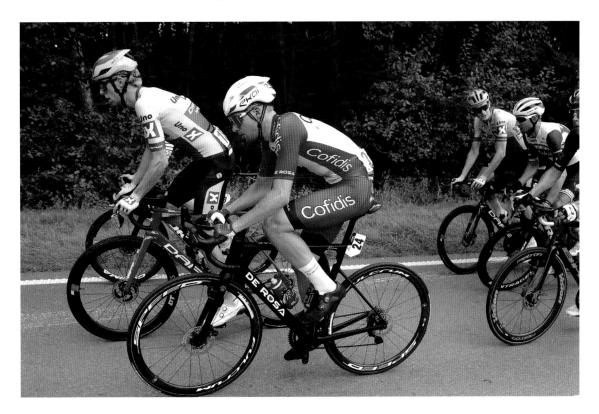

of the hip flexor in comparison to the quad and gluteus maximus is tiny.

This is not to say hip flexors do not give us issues. A cycling posture places us in a predominantly flexed hip, pelvis and lumbar spine position. The hip flexors become used to functioning over a short range of motion. This can lead to their becoming chronically rested in the shortened position, leading to hip pain where they cross and insert, or lower back pain from their origin on the last three lumbar vertebrae, especially when trying to move away from the flexed position (i.e. extending).

Vascular issues

Cyclists are prone to certain vascular issues in and around the hips and pelvis, mainly relating to the iliac arteries that supply blood to the lower limbs. Damage or disease causes the arteries to stretch, narrow and kink in such a way that during high-intensity exercise the blood flow to the affected leg is constricted or obstructed. The lack of blood flow causes pain, burning and/or weakness during cycling and is often noticed as

an unexplained drop in power.

It seems a combination of factors that cycling brings to bear on the iliac arteries is to blame for this. Research tends to agree now that an extremely high blood flow, repetitive hip flexion and closed hip angle (associated with a more aerodynamic position) are the main contributing factors. The resultant continuous, repetitive flexing of the artery under pressure damages the various layers of the artery wall and may stretch or kink it. The artery wall sometimes narrows in response to these changes, a process known as 'endofibrosis'. This means the artery cannot dilate as much during exercise and the result is decreased blood flow to the leg during high intensity cycling.

If you experience the symptoms mentioned – pain or burning within the hip or an unexplained loss in power – in either one or both legs, but only while cycling at high intensity, accurate diagnosis is needed as the condition is often misdiagnosed and mishandled.

This condition, if untreated, can develop to a point where only stopping cycling altogether alleviates

▶ Constricted blood flow in the iliac arteries

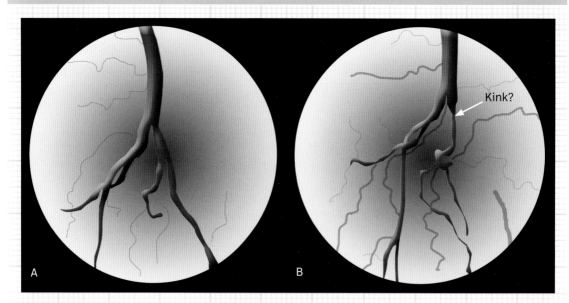

See the difference in blood flow into the smaller arteries from the main trunk artery in B compared to A.
The arrow indicates where the restriction is occuring — probably a kink.

the symptoms and has ended many an aspiring racing cyclist's career. There are several invasive and non-invasive investigations that can help establish the condition's presence. Seek the help of an appropriately qualified medical professional. Surgery to stent the artery walls with plastic tubing or remove a section of the wall is drastic and outcomes are mixed to say the least, so avoid it all costs if possible.

Early diagnosis is essential as changes to the arterial walls are largely permanent. Opening up the hip angle by altering bike position can reduce the stretching and kinking of the arteries as the hip closes and opens. This is why I recommend maintaining an angle of no more than 35-40 degrees when positioning people in aerodynamic time trial or triathlon positions, as avoidance is the best cure for this condition.

Again, shortening crank length can have a huge impact in this area as it can significantly open up the hips. Every 2.5mm drop in crank length can open up your hips by two degrees, so going from 175mm to 165mm is going to potentially have a huge impact.

▶ Hip issues

SOURCE	CAUSE	SOLUTION
Hips – pain or vascular issues	Too closed a hip angle – torso or back angle too low	Adjust reach and drop to relax back angle – opens hip up at same time
	Crank length too long*	Reduce to open hip up
	Cleats too far forward	Closes hip up on back stroke/pull up – adjust
	Leg length difference	Lower longer leg saddle height – closes hip up
	Saddle too low	Raise to open hip
	Saddle too far back	Move forward to open angle up

*This should be your go-to for any hip issues and most bike fit issues.

▶ A closed hip position

See how the hip angle is a lot more closed in B than in A. This is associated with an aerodynamic riding style. Note the knee's proximity to the chest. Too closed a hip angle represents a health risk for some riders due to vascular (blood flow) issues that appear as a sudden loss of power or periodic pain/numbness.

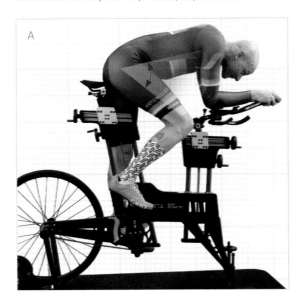
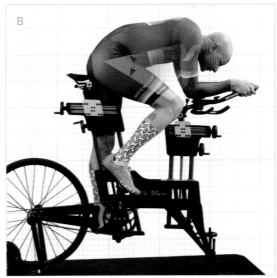

A

B

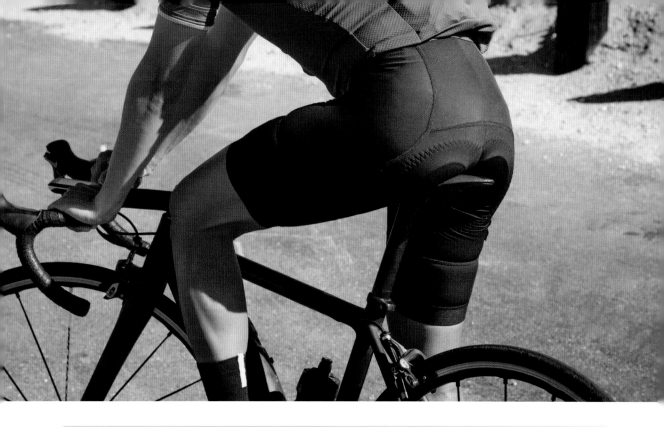

▶ The pelvis interacting with the saddle

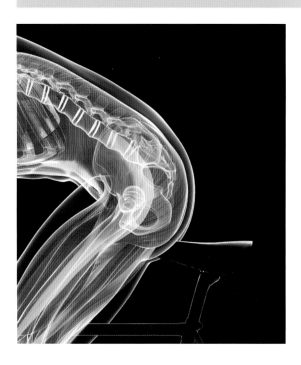

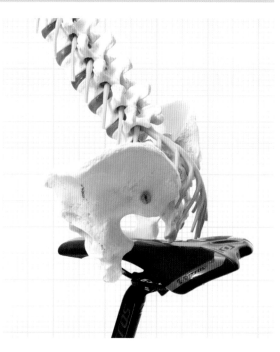

Saddle health

Saddle health issues, which a lot of riders, especially women, suffer from in silence under the misconception that's it's just part of cycling, are very preventable. I'm really proud of the work I did in this area during my time at British Cycling and I am continuing my fight for greater awareness and prevention of this painful barrier to cycling in much of the product development work I'm now involved in.

Saddle soreness vs saddle sores

The first thing to do is differentiate between saddle soreness and saddle sores. Saddle soreness is pain, discomfort and even inflammation that is felt in the areas of your body in contact with the saddle. These can be your sit-bones or, in the case of most riding positions, your perineum. What's important to remember is that your perineum didn't evolve to be sat on and to bear a significant proportion of your body weight for hours! It's also possible to suffer from chafing of your inner thighs as they rub back and forth against

the saddle, but if this is the case, you should be looking for a narrower-nosed saddle.

Mild inflammation and a reddening of the skin can just be an inevitable consequence of a long day in the saddle, can calm down overnight and will occur less as your body gets use to riding. I've already mentioned how stronger riders will tend to suffer less from discomfort as a higher proportion of their weight will be going through their pedals. Also, it's often on really easy-paced recovery spins, when you're barely pressing on your pedals, that soreness can be more of an issue than when you're really pushing hard.

Saddle sores are a physical development of this skin trauma and breakdown, and occur when things go a bit further and get a lot more unpleasant. Folliculitis is an inflammation or infection of the base of a hair follicle, whereas a furuncle is a good old-fashioned boil. Folliculitis is usually pretty painless and tends to clear up, but a boil, if untreated, can grow, become horrendously painful and can keep you off your bike for a long time.

Another unpleasant development can be ulceration. Even the smallest lesion can become ulcerated. With

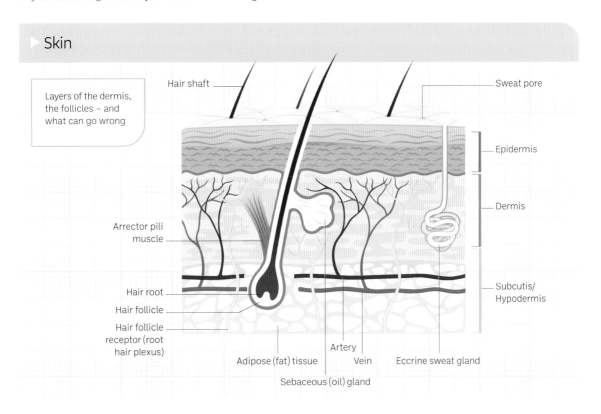

Skin

Layers of the dermis, the follicles – and what can go wrong

Hair shaft

Sweat pore

Epidermis

Dermis

Arrector pili muscle

Subcutis/ Hypodermis

Hair root

Hair follicle

Hair follicle receptor (root hair plexus)

Adipose (fat) tissue

Artery

Vein

Eccrine sweat gland

Sebaceous (oil) gland

It started with a saddle

In the lead up to London 2012, with the UK Institute of Sport, I developed a special saddle for Victoria Pendleton, who'd been suffering from saddle issues that were having a negative impact on her ability to train and her performance. Working on this saddle, in which we used the same silicon rubber as used for breast implants, and solving Victoria's issues really got me thinking about saddle health, specifically for female riders.

After the Games, I wondered how big a problem it was and whether I'd only uncovered the tip of the iceberg. I put together a team and decided to interview riders as part of a qualitative study. The findings were staggering – 100 per cent of the female riders I interviewed were having problems, but, with a male doctor, physio and predominately male coaching staff, didn't feel comfortable mentioning it.

Something had to be done, so I put together a conference of world-class experts. I had tribologists (friction experts), reconstructive surgeons, who were experts in dealing with pressure sores, and a top consultant in vulval health.

I then produced full care instructions for all the riders and focused on developing saddle technology and kit. This significantly improved saddle health, and reduced saddle discomfort and injuries across the entire team.

It was during this time I also started to notice that, especially with aggressive pursuiting positions, the UCI's ruling that saddles have to be level was a definite contributing factor to some of the issues that female riders on the squad were having. I could see no logical reason for the rule and took my concerns to them. Once they were aware that their ruling could be having damaging health implications for riders and could expose them from a legal perspective, they quickly looked to amend the rule. They consulted with me for my recommendations regarding tilt and the rulebook was changed. To have actually altered the rules of the sport that I was working in, especially as the change will benefit the health of riders, is something I'm really proud of.

▶ Cutaway saddles

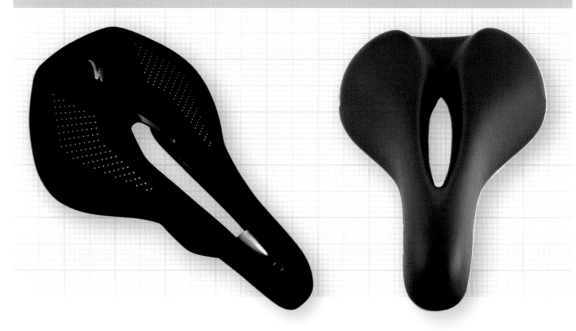

the outer layer of skin gone, bacteria can get into the deeper layers where they thrive in the warm and damp environment. If untreated, the ulcer will grow and can lead to a serious skin infection.

Female riders have to contend with labial swelling and grazing that, if ignored, can become extremely painful and serious. Issues specific to male riders include penile numbness due to pressure on the pudendal nerve that, if ignored, can lead to the development of erectile dysfunction.

WHY DOES IT HAPPEN?

There are four main factors that contribute to skin breakdown and the development of saddle soreness and sores.

Pressure: When sat on a saddle, much of your body weight is focused on a tiny area, resulting in immense pressure. This compresses underlying structures such as capillaries, reducing blood flow.

Shear/friction: Every pedal stroke you make results in a slight shift of weight, causing you to move from side to side on your saddle. This builds heat via friction and soon results in soreness and abrasions. Shear also compounds the effect of pressure, further reducing blood flow.

Moisture: The moisture from sweating results in an increase in shear.

Temperature: As you ride, skin temperature, particularly of your perineum, rises. This raises skin metabolism, but, as a result of pressure and shear, blood flow is severely reduced, meaning the skin doesn't get the oxygen and nutrients it needs to function effectively and it begins to break down.

PREVENTING SADDLE SORENESS AND SORES

As with all sports injuries, prevention is the best cure. Don't wait until you have a problem in this area, take steps to prevent it, because once it does become an issue, it's almost guaranteed to cost you time on the bike. I worked with one rider who, having had a really nasty walnut-sized infection after getting a graze from a poorly fitted skin suit, had a repeat of the same painful condition a year later. The problem was that the infection had literally carved out a cavity in his dermis that would then always be a higher risk area for problems. Both incidents each cost him four weeks off the bike, courses

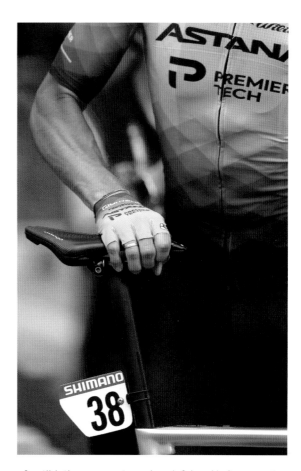

of antibiotics, were extremely painful and he's now got to be super-careful to avoid more problems in the future.

BIKE FIT AND SADDLE CHOICE

If you're experiencing unusual levels of saddle discomfort on the bike, always go back to the fundamentals of saddle height, fore/aft position and tilt. If you notice that soreness tends to be worse on one side than the other, this can be an indicator of leg length discrepancy. Once you are confident that your position is right, work through the steps described earlier to help you identify the right saddle for you.

STRUCTURED TRAINING

By following a structured training plan and building up your time in the saddle gradually, your body and backside do seem to adapt and 'toughen up'. Suddenly upping your mileage is a guaranteed route to soreness. As previously mentioned, as you get stronger, you'll also put proportionally more weight through your pedals than your backside.

STAND UP

Even on flat rides, get into the habit of standing out of the saddle every five to 10 minutes to ease pressure and restore blood flow. This is also really important when you're doing turbo sessions.

SHORTS AND CHAMOIS

In the same way that saddle choice is highly personal, so is finding the best shorts and chamois for you. Don't think that spending more guarantees a blissful ride because if the chamois is in the wrong place for you, or the fit isn't quite right or there's a seam that rubs, even the most expensive shorts on the market won't do the job.

The chamois, or, more accurately, pad, needs to follow similar width guidelines as when choosing a saddle. Look for one that matches your sit-bone width and go from there. Currently the go-to material for pads is foam as this does a great job of wicking away sweat. However, this is indicative of almost all the main pad

manufactures being based in Italy, where it's hot. For most riders, prioritising dealing with pressure and friction would yield better results. I'm currently working on a pad with Endura using medical grade silicon embedded in the foam to achieve this, and the next step will be to use a silicon foam that will deliver top wicking performance, too. I'm also pressing for a range of chamois widths to be available. I believe it's going to be a while before the saddle industry delivers a wide enough range of female-specific saddles, but at least we can try to produce a range of pads to try to compensate for this a bit.

Make sure your shorts fit well and that the pad is long enough and where it should be, especially when you're bent forward in your riding position. Shorts also need to have decent grippers around the thigh to stop them riding up. You also need to make sure that they're tight enough to hold the pad in place, but not so tight as to be restrictive to movement. Check that there are no badly placed seams. When working with Team Sky we had to change Ian Stannard's saddle to one with a cut-out as the sponsor-supplied shorts had a seam on the

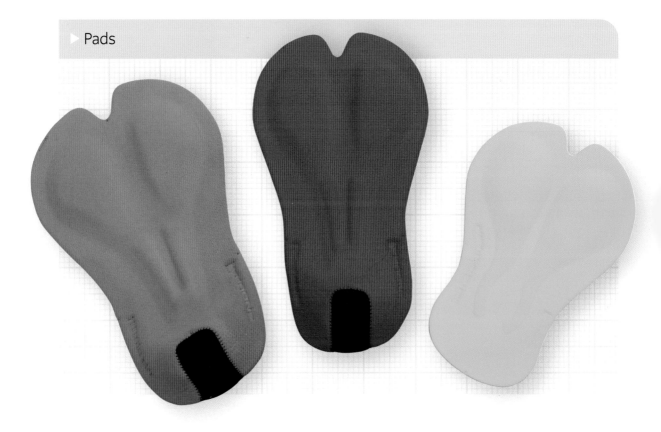

▶ Pads

pad that was causing him some very painful chaffing in a very sensitive area! Another example of a change in pad causing problems was when GB's track riders had to wear white Leaders skin suits in the UCI World Cup. They caused problems throughout the squad, but especially for our female team pursuiters, and we ended up cutting out the pads and getting our own sewn in.

CHAMOIS CREAM

I find it unbelievable that there are cyclists who don't use chamois cream. Prevention is always better than cure and, even if you've never suffered from any saddle discomfort, for such a simple, inexpensive but effective preventative step, it's a no-brainer. Chamois cream works by reducing friction and acting as a barrier to protect the skin and maintain an optimal hydration level – not too wet and not too dry. I've developed a pre- and post-ride system that comprises of a highly effective barrier cream for on the bike, a wash that removes the oils in the chamois cream from your skin but leaves your natural oils, and finally a super-hydrating and soothing moisturiser.

SELF-CARE AND HYGIENE

A common mistake a lot of new cyclists make is to wear underwear with cycling shorts. Never do this, especially with cotton underwear, as it will hold moisture next to your skin, negating the wicking effect of quality shorts and pad, and increasing the likelihood of soreness and infection.

When you get back from your ride or finish a turbo session, don't sit around sipping coffee and checking out your stats on Strava in your damp and sweaty shorts. Get them off, get clean and then relax.

In the shower, make sure you clean thoroughly but don't scrub and avoid using flannels, sponges and exfoliators. Avoid removing all the natural oils and bacteria, which both enhance the barrier function of the epidermis. Use a gentle washing cream, such as the one I've developed, or something like Dermol 500, and always rinse well with plenty of plain water. Pat dry and avoid rubbing. Wear loose clothing to aid drying and airflow. Use an unperfumed moisturiser to improve barrier function and to soothe any inflammation.

Probably more applicable to female cyclists, but,

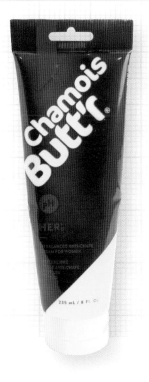

Chamois cream

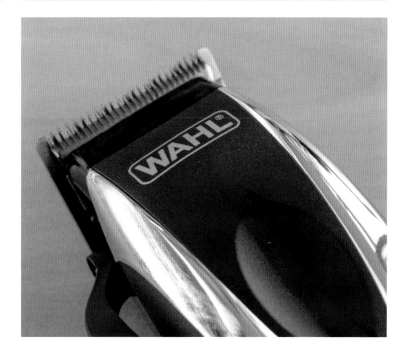

Clippers

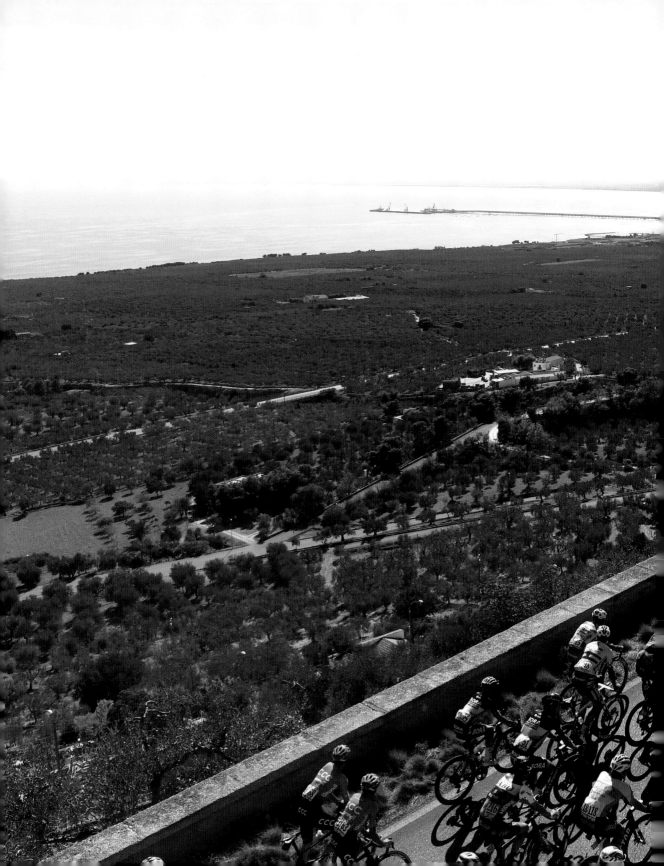

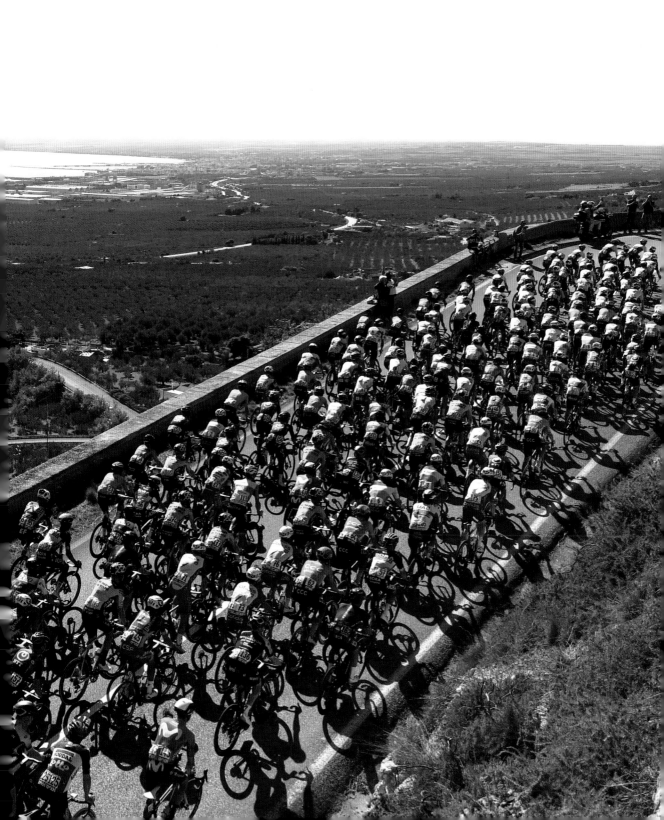

in these days of 'manscaping', for the guys too, clip rather than shave. Hair provides some protection from friction and shaving, and as well as irritating the skin, shaving can also lead to ingrowing hairs and folliculitis. If you do need to tidy down there, opt for clippers.

Lower back pain

Lower back pain is a common complaint among cyclists. It is rarely bad enough to stop people completely, but studies of both professional and non-competitive cyclists have shown lower back pain causes the highest rates of functional impairment and people seeking medical attention.

It should, of course, be noted that many people already have a back issue not caused by cycling, which riding can either alleviate or make worse. Cycling remains a great way of getting cardiovascular exercise without pain or injury due to its low-impact nature.

If the causes of lower back pain in cycling can be identified and treated, or avoided, then cycling actually represents one of the best ways to exercise for people with chronic back pain. Causes of lower back pain can be activity-related or equipment-related.

ACTIVITY-RELATED

Activity-related causes include sudden increases in distances, loads or intensity, for example climbing long hills or mountains for the first time. If you suspect these may be the reason for your back pain, consider stepping back a little in terms of activity and building up more slowly. If given time, the body will adapt to the imposed demand or load – if it can.

EQUIPMENT-RELATED

Equipment-related causes include saddle height, saddle angle, and drop and reach. With the saddle too high the rider rocks from side to side trying to reach the pedals with each stroke. Bilateral saddle soreness often accompanies back pain caused in this way.

Saddle angle alters the torso angle and has been proven to have a dramatic effect on the relief of lower back pain. In a study of 80 club cyclists, angling their saddle down by 10–15 degrees reduced incidences of lower back

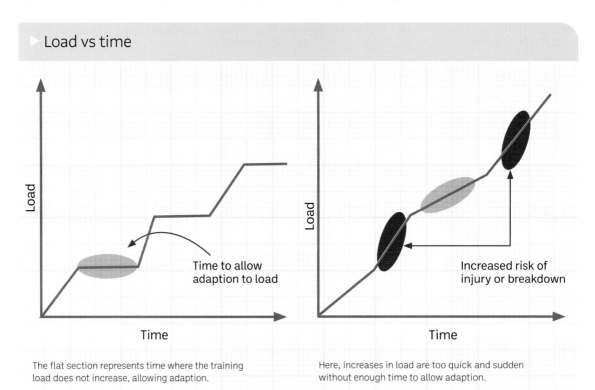

▶ Load vs time

Load (y-axis) / **Time** (x-axis)

Time to allow adaption to load

The flat section represents time where the training load does not increase, allowing adaption.

Load (y-axis) / **Time** (x-axis)

Increased risk of injury or breakdown

Here, increases in load are too quick and sudden without enough time to allow adaption.

pain by 72 per cent while cycling over six months.

If reach is too great it forces the rider's body to flex further from the lower back and creates an acute torso angle. A sustained, excessively flexed posture can cause pain over time. People with tight hamstrings are more predisposed to this type of lower back pain as the pelvis is held back by the hamstrings pulling on it, forcing the lower back to flex more in order to reach the handlebars.

In bike-fitting terms excessive drop and/or reach is seen in the angle of the torso. This is the angle formed by the horizontal plane of the hips/pelvis to the line of the torso. Recreational road riders have an angle of between 45 and 50 degrees, while pros can get to 35 degrees, and a good time-trial position is as low as 20 degrees.

Remember that drop and reach are a function of saddle height and angle, top tube length, stem length and steerer tube height.

The easiest way to address excessive drop is to relax the front end of the bike fit by raising the handlebars, which of course shortens the reach (the head tube is angled rearwards, remember) as well. Excessive reach

can be adjusted by altering the stem length or saddle fore/aft. Be careful with the latter as it has implications for the whole rear end set-up. Unless the saddle is identified as excessively rearwards I would always shorten the stem first to address excessive reach. As a general rule, however, a stem of less than 90mm starts to affect the handling of the bike and if you feel you need to set it this long it is a clear indication that the top tube and therefore the bike frame is the wrong size for you.

An aggressive position of the kind that is often perceived as aerodynamic, with a lot of drop and reach, is a common cause of cyclists' lower back pain. In my experience, a position like this takes time to adapt to. Start from the sustainable position in which you can ride without discomfort, then make gradual adjustments towards your goal, allowing the body time to adapt. Often, combining this with a flexibility programme targeted to your limiting factors – say tight hamstrings – will pay dividends.

A great way to look at pain and dysfunction, and to make sense of it, is to consider this. We are all ageing and wearing out little by little; life is finite. Compare

Back angles

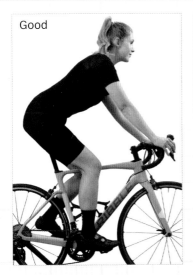

Good

A balanced position, having an evenly flexed spine with good weight distribution.

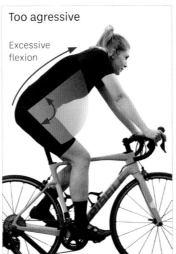

Too agressive

Excessive flexion

The excessive drop and reach and the rider's tight hamstrings holding her pelvis back result in excessive lumbar flexion.

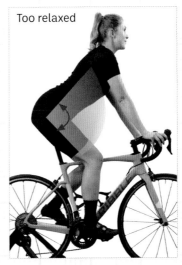

Too relaxed

You can be too relaxed. The high front end has forced the rider to sit up, leaving too much weight through her back.

two people with identical degenerative lower back conditions. One has pain and one has none. Why? They have the same pathology? Pain and dysfunction, it turns out, do not correlate well. One explanation is that the body only complains when it cannot cope or keep up with the level and amount of degeneration, i.e. when it is occurring too quickly.

At one end of the spectrum, a crash and fractured collarbone is an immediately traumatic assault on the body, which causes a lot of pain. At the other end, a degenerative lumbar spine segment – disc and bone – may just need time to adapt (ligaments lengthen, nerves glide more smoothly, scar tissue modifies) to a sustained flexed position.

A very successful road rider came to see me years ago when he was part of the British Cycling Academy. He'd always suffered back pain on long mountain climbs. He wanted to know if there was anything that could be done in the long term to the way his body worked that could help him. I explained to him that we could help by making him more able to cope with the demands of mountain climbing, but possibly at the expense of his

sprint. He took one look at me and said he'd live with the pain. Just as Usain Bolt couldn't win a marathon, this rider was built for speed and power, and these characteristics do not lend themselves to coping with long, sustained climbing without pain.

INTRINSIC FACTORS

Intrinsic factors are those relating to the way your body is. They include different leg lengths, poor flexibility, saddle injury and previous lumbar spine injuries.

When poor flexibility and bad bike position meet, quite often it is the lower back that bears the burden of the problem. As discussed earlier in the section on reach, the posterior chain – muscles down your back – needs to be flexible enough for the position you have set. If it is not, you should relax the position, usually by raising the front end, until the muscles have adapted. Riding a very slightly lower position week by week, month by month may be sufficient to achieve your goal, but you may have to work off the bike to achieve your best level of flexibility. A saddle injury can lead to back pain as the rider tries to alleviate the pressure of sitting on the sore

▶ Leg length difference

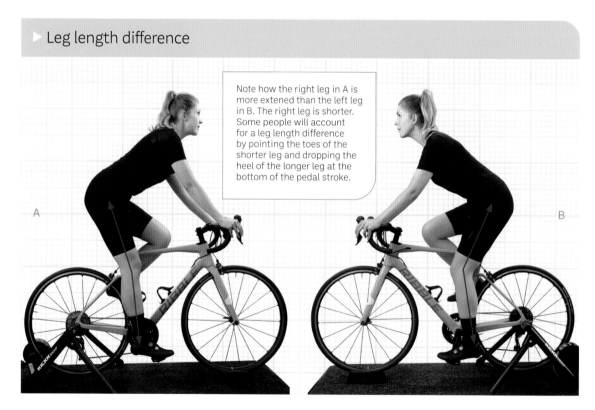

Note how the right leg in A is more extended than the left leg in B. The right leg is shorter. Some people will account for a leg length difference by pointing the toes of the shorter leg and dropping the heel of the longer leg at the bottom of the pedal stroke.

A

B

area and so compromises the lower back. More often than not the sore will be unilateral or to one side.

Leg length difference

Human beings are not symmetrical. Asymmetry is the norm and this can be the source of problems when we interact with symmetrical, fixed equipment, such as a bike.

A difference in the length of one of your lower limbs, whether it be structural (actual longer bones) or functional (twists in the pelvis and surrounding soft tissues that make a limb seem shorter), presents an asymmetry that the body must absorb, because the distance to the pedals remains the same. In my experience, actual leg length differences (LLD) are pretty rare, but functional ones are relatively common. A significant LLD – more than 3mm – has to be accommodated while riding. Many do so without ever realising it. Plenty, however, do not.

So how do you know if you have LLD? The best way to identify structural LLD is to use a scannogram that takes a large X-ray picture of your whole lower body. Radiologists can then measure the length of the bones. However, this method has it flaws and is only 75–85 per cent accurate. It will not, of course, show a functional LLD that occurs when your body twists when moving.

A definitive diagnosis needs to be built up from layers of information. With each relevant symptom or sign the weight of possibility increases that someone has an LLD that requires intervention.

Clues

Unilateral saddle soreness: persistent one-sided saddle soreness is suggestive of a rider sitting predominantly to one side of the saddle, and one reason for doing this is in order to make a shorter leg reach the pedal.

One knee tracks differently: one knee tracks in a much wider elliptical fashion than the other, which is more piston-like (going straight up and down). A rider may well unknowingly set their saddle height in favour of their shorter leg, which will take the most direct path to reach the pedal, leaving the other leg to compensate with elliptical tracking.

One-sided back pain: the twist or rotation through three planes the pelvis has to do to accommodate a significant LLD often means the base of the spine – the

▶ Scannogram

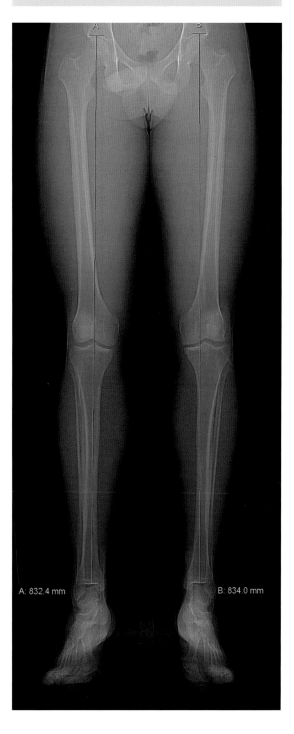

A: 832.4 mm   B: 834.0 mm

▶ Pelvic rocking due to LLD

You often see rocking of the plevis from side to side when the sadlle is too high. If someone has a leg length difference the saddle is too high on one side so they only rock one way.

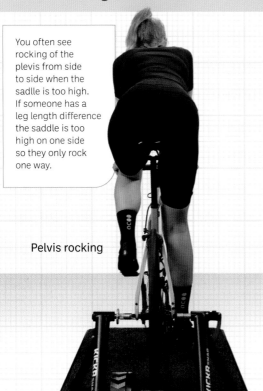

Pelvis rocking

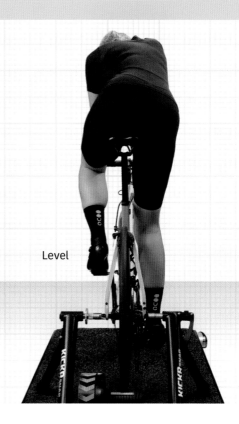

Level

▶ Lower back issues

SOURCE	CAUSE	SOLUTION
Lower back pain	Torso or back angle too low – too much reach	Reduce reach – shorten stem, move saddle forward if knee not compromised
	Torso or back angle too low – too much drop	Raise handlebars, drop saddle if knee angle allows
	Both of the above	Shorten stem, raise handlebars and, if knee movement allows, drop saddle and move it forward
	Leg length difference	Adjust saddle height to optimal for long leg and accommodate shorter one by building up
	Saddle choice	If the saddle blocks pelvic rotation it can force lower back to flex more – different shaped saddles help
	Nose-up	Nose-up saddles forces pelvis backwards increasing flexion and strain on lower back

sacrum – is offset and under pressure. The lumbar spine, or lower back, sits on top of this and, like any structure, if the foundation isn't optimal problems can follow.

Calf strain or tightness: often the shorter leg will adopt a more ankling pedalling style, much more toes-down at BDC and heel-down at TDC. Once again, this is so the shorter leg can reach the pedals.

One-sided knee pain: if this cannot be explained by any other means, it may be due to one knee failing to cope with the body's adaptive changes to LLD. For example, the adaptive rotation of the pelvis either backwards or forward (anterior or posterior rotation) effectively changes the knee forward of foot setting.

> When one of British Cycling's Olympic Team Pursuit gold medallists first started cycling, she repeatedly pulled or strained her left calf. Investigations showed a significantly shorter leg on that side. Correction of the problem, the placement of a 6mm shim under her left cleat, saw it disappear.

Shoulders

The most common problem cyclists experience in the shoulder area is a fractured collarbone from a crash. On the bike, however, issues relating to bike fit are often secondary in severity and nature at the shoulder compared to other areas, though they are still linked.

Someone who has too much weight on their hands may well notice numbness in that area first (see page 134), but this can also be associated with pain in the shoulder or shoulder blades. If the body weight is pushed forward, it can force the elbows to straighten or lock out, shifting the attenuation and control of the upper limbs solely to the shoulder. During long rides this may result in the slow, gradual build-up of achy, burning pain between the shoulder blades or at the back of the shoulder. So look for a combination of the following: numbness in the hands, elbows locked, duration-related pain in the shoulder blades. All these symptoms point to a position in which too much weight is being placed on the handlebars. Consequently, this can be corrected by raising the front end of the bike.

Incorrect handlebar width, both too narrow and too wide, can also lead to shoulder pain. Your thumbs and fingers on the hoods should be in line with the outside of your shoulder and this is easy to check in a mirror.

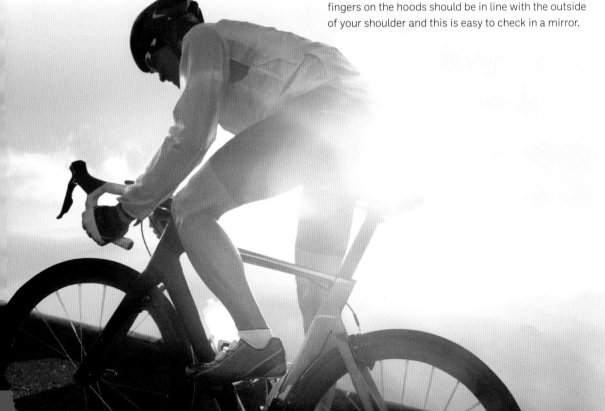

Too wide, too narrow and correct bars

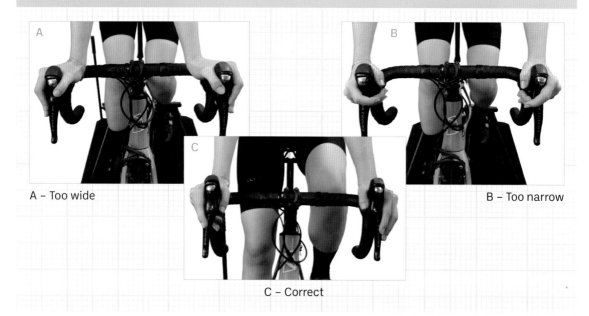

A – Too wide

C – Correct

B – Too narrow

Shoulder pain

Note the forward protracted position (reaching) of the rider's shoulder and the locked-out elbows and wrists, causing all force to go to the shoulder.

locked out arms

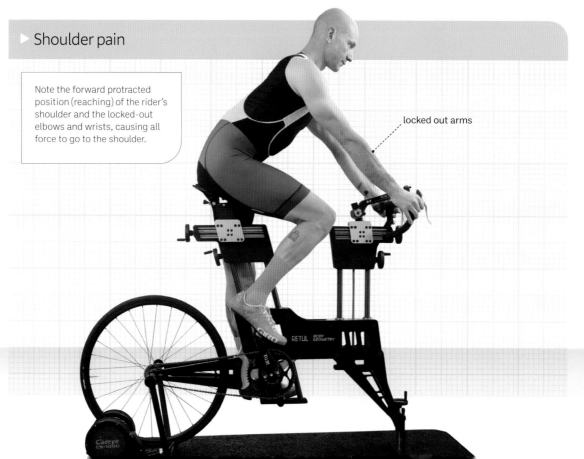

Neck

The neck and upper back play a vital role in cycling: without them we wouldn't be able to extend our heads into position to see forward. Problems occur when you have to extend your neck a lot to achieve this basic requirement. Excessive handlebar drop is the most common cause of neck pain, the low torso angle created having to be countered by an equal amount of neck craning.

The neck musculature in a cyclist adapts to cope with the demands of postural endurance – hours in the same position holding the head up. This is a very different set of demands compared to, for example, a rugby prop forward or an NFL linebacker. People increasing the duration of their riding quickly experience postural neck pain as the muscles struggle to cope with the new demands placed on them. Indeed, ultra-distance cyclists in the Race Across America suffer terribly with debilitating neck pain – often referred to as Shermer's neck after one of the most famous riders in this hardest of events. People have even devised neck braces to alleviate the work done by the neck muscles in ultra-distance cycling. It is strange to think it's the neck that can stop someone's race long before their legs, heart or lungs.

In my off-the-bike routine I include work on the cervical area and, along with the step of raising the front end of the bike, if you do suffer from neck pain, this can be very effective.

LOW HANDLEBARS CAUSING NECK PAIN

The eyes have to look up the road. To achieve this the neck has to extend to lift the head. If the drop and reach are excessive the neck has to extend even further. This can cause pain and discomfort on long rides.

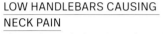

Neck pain

Neck braces

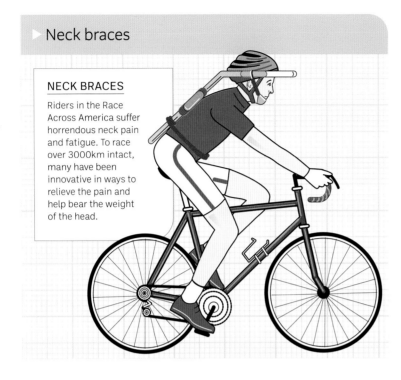

NECK BRACES

Riders in the Race Across America suffer horrendous neck pain and fatigue. To race over 3000km intact, many have been innovative in ways to relieve the pain and help bear the weight of the head.

Upper limb pain

SOURCE	CAUSE	SOLUTION
Overworked or painful shoulders, elbows or hands	Too much reach	Reduce reach to relax straight elbows and protracted shoulders
	Too much drop	Reduce weight on hands, elbows, shoulders by raising handlebars
	Saddle tilted forward	Level saddle to reduce pelvis being tipped forward and all rider's weight onto hands
Hand and forearm pain	Hand position on bars too wide/ narrow handlebars	Adjust to fit your shoulder width
	Hoods rotated too far forward	Move around handlebars
	Narrow girth of bars	Double bar tape reduces not only vibration but allows more open grip of the bar with the hand

Triceps

The triceps – like most of the upper body's musculature – act as attenuators, absorbing the demands of a sustained posture and the vibrations or shocks from the road. Most people notice some triceps fatigue-related pain as they start to ride longer and longer. If the pain persists, however, re-examine the load being placed through your arms by your position. If you're riding with your arms fully locked out all the time, your triceps are inevitably going to fatigue and you should recheck your reach.

Hands and fingers

Some cycling ailments are confined to the elite and some to recreational riders. I don't think I saw a single rider during my time at British Cycling with numb or tingling hands. However, I have seen serious recreational cyclists with quite debilitating hand-nerve injuries referred to me by local doctors.

The ulnar nerve is the most commonly injured, followed by the median. These nerves pass close to the surface in and around the wrist and palm, and are constrained by structures around them. This means that they can become compressed when sustained pressure is applied – for example, when resting the palm of your hand on the handlebar or brake hoods during long rides. The nerves supply sensation and power to the hand and finger muscles; compression alters or blocks these, leading to numbness, pins and needles, and even weakness.

The most common distribution or pattern of these symptoms is to the little or ring fingers, as these are the areas supplied by the ulnar nerve. Symptoms in the thumb and index finger point to median nerve compression.

In milder cases the vibrations from the road up through the bike can be enough to cause symptoms. Interventions such as double bar tape, bar gels and mitts with gel padding can really help this.

If there is too much weight being borne by the upper limbs and ultimately the palm of the hands, your position holds the key. Raising your handlebars and shortening the reach can help reduce the load on your hands. Check your saddle is not pointing nose down. This has the effect of tipping the rider onto the handlebars from the pelvis, creating pressure on the hands as the upper limbs lock out and attempt to push back.

Beware

I was asked to consult on a local businessman's total ulnar neuropathy (an injury where the ulnar nerve is irreversibly damaged). He had recently ridden the Lands End–John O'Groats. A poor bike fit beforehand had lured him into thinking he was OK to carry on with numb hands and that this was just part of long-distance cycling. He had been wrongly positioned with so much weight on his hands that over the course of the ride he compressed his ulnar nerve to such an extent that he caused permanent damage, leaving him with loss of sensation over his little and ring finger. It's perfectly acceptable to experience transient, occasional numbness or pins and needles on long rides, but persistent or constant symptoms like these need further attention and investigation.

▶ Compression areas in the hand

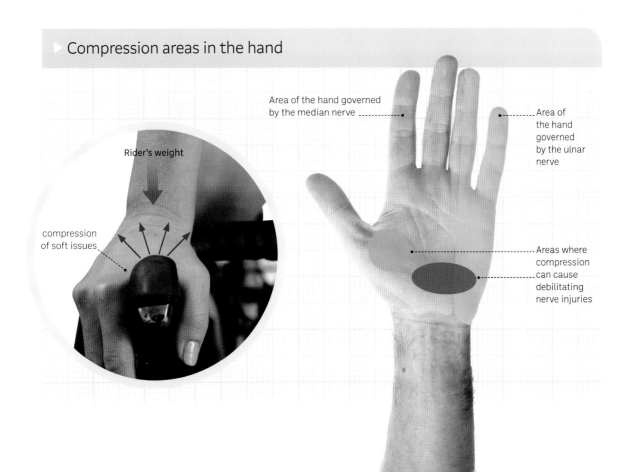

Rider's weight

compression of soft issues

Area of the hand governed by the median nerve

Area of the hand governed by the ulnar nerve

Areas where compression can cause debilitating nerve injuries

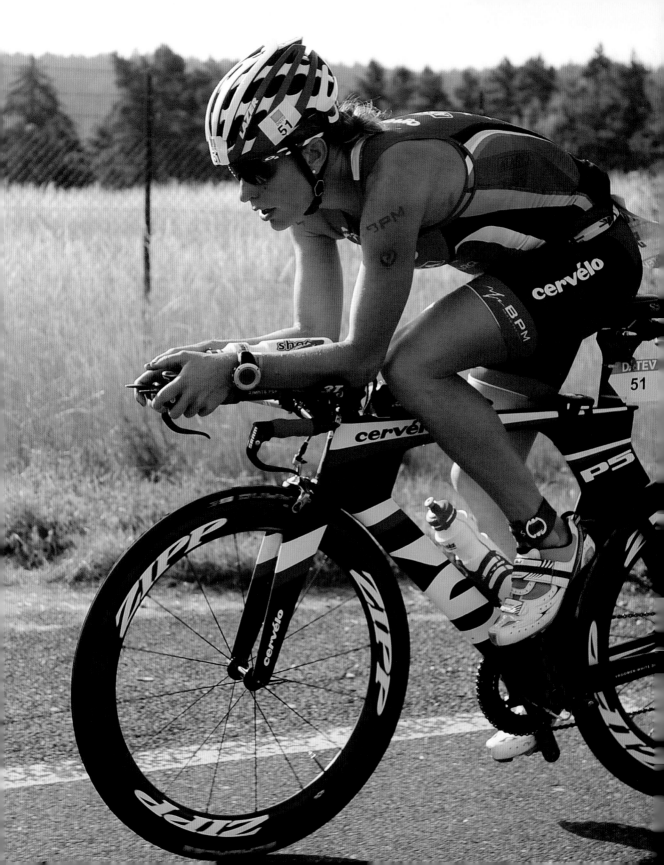

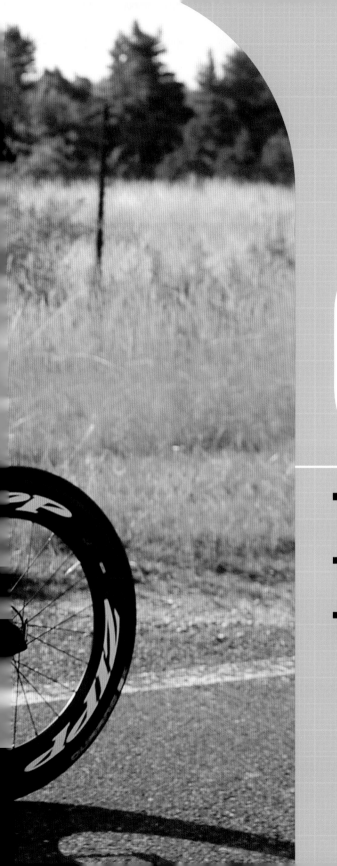

06

Time trial and triathlon

Time trial and triathlon

Since leaving British Cycling, I've worked with a huge number of cyclists across almost all disciplines. A lot of these are time triallists who, because the aerodynamics pillar is the main factor and the kit is different to road riding, need more detailed advice.

I'm also now working with a lot of triathletes, including GB Triathlon, and in non-drafting events, including Ironman distance racing, aerodynamics is also key. Triathlon is so exciting to work in, because without the restrictions on bike design and rider position imposed by the UCI, you can really push the limits.

Aerodynamics

When trying to go fast on a bike, your biggest enemy to overcome is air resistance and, although riders obsess about wheels, frame profiling and hidden cables, their impact is minimal compared to the drag created by the fleshy lump sat on top of the bike. In cycling disciplines against the clock, such as time trials and pursuit, and ever more so on the road, aero is king and I'm seeing more and more amateur riders who are looking to make their position as slippery as possible.

My early understanding of aerodynamics came about by spending time with Chris Boardman and Matt Parker (Head of Marginal Gains at British Cycling and the brains of the Secret Squirrel Club). It was my job to 'close the loop' after a rider had been to a wind tunnel positional session: to understand a potential new position and advise whether it was achievable or what had to happen to make it so. A good aero position for the team pursuit or time trial has to be worked at and evolved, be it suffering time in the position to get used to it, or stretching and strengthening in order to hold it.

Why is it so important? Apart from on steep inclines, nearly 80 per cent of a rider's energy goes into forcing the air in front of him or her out of the way.

That's why cyclists obsess about being aero. If you can reduce the amount of air you are pushing and the energy cost associated with that, you can go further and faster under the same power. But cyclists often look in the wrong place for the biggest and easiest gains to be made in aerodynamics.

If we break down the total contribution to aerodynamic drag, the bike only accounts for 20 per cent and the rider on top of it 80 per cent. Bike aerodynamics are, of course, important, but there are huge gains to be made in the shape and position of the rider. The importance of bike aerodynamics is overplayed, because that is where the commercial interest of bike manufacturers lies – they want to sell you aero kit.

What is aerodynamics? I hate equations, but I think breaking down and understanding this one makes sense if you are going to invest time, effort and possibly money in your aerodynamics:

$D = \frac{1}{2}pCdAv^2$

D – the total aerodynamic drag
p – the air density
Cd – coefficient of drag
A – the rider's frontal surface area or silhouette
V – the cyclist's velocity

The power you require to overcome the aerodynamic drag (D) on a bike is related to the air density (p – how thick the air in front of you is; a higher altitude means thinner air), frontal area (A – are you a 'brick or a blade',? as coaches like to say), your drag coefficient

(Cd – how the air flows around you, determined by your shape and surface) and speed. Rider position changes concerned with aerodynamics are aimed at reducing the frontal area and optimising how the air flows over the rider, measured by the Cd or coefficient of drag. Drag for riders is multifactorial: air that becomes disturbed behind a rider's head or helmet isn't flowing as quickly as the air in front over the smooth helmet. This creates a pressure difference and therefore drag, with the slower-moving air almost sucking or dragging the rider back.

It's the same principle as the Venturi effect responsible for flight, which uses the same forces to create uplift instead of drag. Unfortunately, riders, unlike wings, are complicated shapes – all tubes and cylinders – of infinitely varying sizes. I think this is why researchers have struggled to establish linear relationships between frontal area and drag: the human body is just so differently shaped and the science of computational fluid dynamics so complicated that a package that is more aero for one rider may well not be for another.

Aero testing

Aero testing has definitely become more accessible and affordable to all cyclists and, whether it's time in the wind tunnel, velodrome testing with systems such as Alphamantis or green screen testing using the Bioracer system, it's no longer the preserve of elite athletes.

However, although it might now be easier to find your optimal aerodynamic position, it's likely that that position won't be suitable for you at that moment. Go to any triathlon, especially long course, and you'll see athletes with super-aggressive set-ups who are riding a significant proportion of the bike leg sat upright on their bull-horns, because they're unable to hold the position the wind tunnels set for them.

If we go back to the fundamentals of bike fit and the three pillars of aerodynamics, power production and sustainability/comfort, for longer time trials and triathlon bike legs, yes, optimising aerodynamics is important, but not with a disregard for sustainability.

When I was at British Cycling, riders almost had to earn the right to go to the wind tunnel. They had to demonstrate that they had the range of movement in

▶ **Aerodynamics**

AIRFLOW OVER A RIDER

Note the turbulence behind the head.

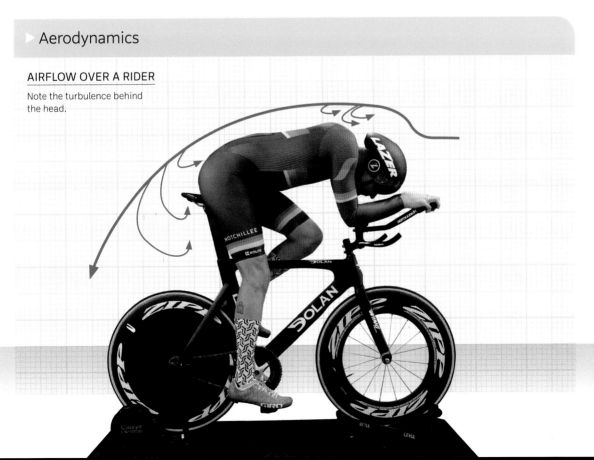

their hamstrings, thoracic spine, lats and neck, so that their body wouldn't be a limiting factor when they got in the tunnel.

The position that aero testing gives you is likely to be at the extreme end of your fit window, a gold standard and, for the majority of riders, will take a lot of time and effort to adapt to.

Even though we are focusing here on positional changes, it's worth noting that what surrounds that position is also very important, for example clothing. Surround the best aero position with a baggy T-shirt and shorts, and the guy with a less efficient position, but wearing a good skin suit and helmet will go faster. The interaction between the materials we wear and the air flowing over us makes a huge difference to drag. I mention the helmet because it makes a big difference in smoothing out the airflow behind your head, which is a major contributor to turbulence and therefore drag.

Chris Boardman's philosophy worked on using the full-length mirror to reduce the frontal area, or silhouette, by manipulating position. If you're starting from scratch, the first and biggest gains to be had are – generally – by getting your shoulders rounded, bringing your elbows in and going lower. I say 'generally' as it is well-established now that for some people there is a point where going lower forces them to pop their head up. The whole idea in being low at the front is to hide the head in front of a flatter torso, making the silhouette of the rider smaller. So if the head pops up, that is counterproductive. This usually boils down to the rider's flexibility in the thoracic spine and shoulders (latissimus dorsi length). Pulling the elbows in works best for smaller riders, allowing air to flow around the body. Bigger riders sometimes benefit from setting the elbow

Three things that generally make you more aero

▶ Rounded shoulders
▶ Elbows in (unless you're over 183cm – then consider wider)
▶ Lower at the front (to a point!)

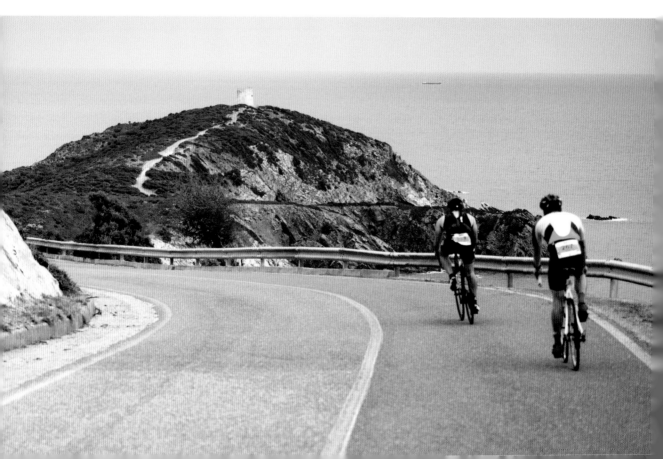

pads on their tri-bars wider to allow air to flow over the chest rather than all the way around.

In trying to achieve this at home, you either need lots of stems and steering tubes of different lengths, or an adjustable stem such as the Look Ergo. This makes adjusting your front end quick and easy, which is essential in allowing you to quickly change between two positions and feel the difference. Feel should not be underestimated. It may not be scientific or objective, but we discard the subjective to our detriment. You, the rider, are the complicated measuring machine: your feedback includes more data than any computer and is important in the evaluation of how a new position will fare.

Chris Boardman has a great way of putting this: 'Cycling is based on the three Ps: Power, Pulse and Perception.' In trying a new position he always has a view to seeing whether he thinks he could work with it over longer trials and training to become sustainable. Sustainable is another key word. An aero position is quite often not comfortable, so we usually change the question on comfort to: is this position sustainable?

If it's so uncomfortable you have to shift around every 20 seconds, disturbing your silhouette as you go forward, it is not sustainable and should be adjusted until it is.

In trying to reduce the silhouette many go for an arms out or longer style, which looks more aero, but in actual fact doesn't reduce the frontal area, and is not as comfortable and efficient as having your elbows at 90 degrees. This is a very effective position in which to bear the upper body's weight when time trialling.

Testing methods

DIY AERO TESTING

Even though aero testing has become more affordable and accessible, for the majority of riders, it's still not a viable option. However, you can definitely check and improve your position at home. Chris Boardman would take head-on photos of himself, cut out his outline, trace this onto graph paper and work out his frontal area from this. You could easily adopt a similar approach using modern photo-editing software.

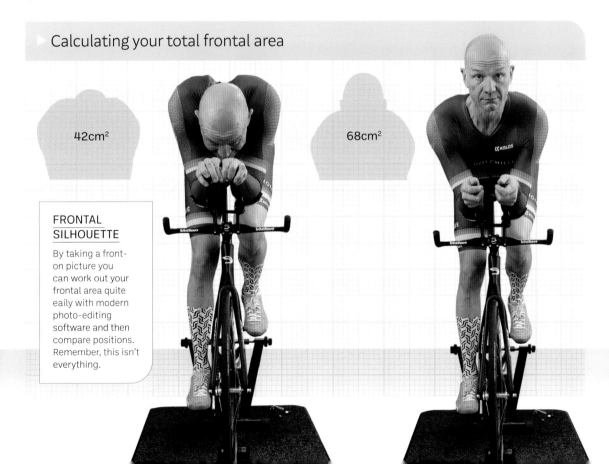

► Calculating your total frontal area

42cm²

68cm²

FRONTAL SILHOUETTE

By taking a front-on picture you can work out your frontal area quite eaily with modern photo-editing software and then compare positions. Remember, this isn't everything.

Indoor trainers are brilliant for working on your aero position. You can take side-on images and videos while you ride, compare your position to top riders, feel how tweaks affect your ability to hold a position and, if you've got a smart trainer or power meter, check the impact on power production.

As general rules of thumb, lower at the front is always going to be faster, so you should be looking to get your back as flat as possible, but by rotating your pelvis forward, facilitated by saddle choice and positioning and ideally shorter cranks, keeping your hip angle open. There is a point, though, where, if you go too low, you'll start sacrificing power and your head will probably pop up. Remember, although you might be able to get into a position on the indoor trainer, holding it on the road and being able to safely handle your bike and see where you're going can be a different matter.

High, in-front-of-the-face 'praying mantis' hand positions are very in vogue at the moment and, regardless of the direct aero gains, with a pelvis

rotated to a forward position it can really help to almost lock you in place and support your position.

Once you've found a position, as I've previously said, you've then got to spend a significant amount of time riding in it so that it becomes sustainable and second nature to you. If your time trial or triathlon position feels odd, unstable, unfamiliar or you can't hold it, it's not correct.

ROLL-DOWN TEST

Find a hill which has an uphill section at the foot of the descent. Roll down it without pedalling and see how far your position allows you to roll up the other side. An obvious issue with this is the weather changing, which can affect the validity and repeatability of tests.

CALCULATING DRAG

There are several websites and even bike gadgets that will allow you to calculate your drag coefficient if you can record several variables: speed, power, air pressure, weight and rolling resistance. Temperature and wind speed need to be controlled for it to be accurate. If you have a power meter then the Aerolab function in the (free) Golden Cheetah software is an accurate way of comparing different positions by riding laps of a circuit.

VELODROME

With all the above data, the last two variables can be controlled much more easily in a velodrome and track testing is much more realistic than a wind tunnel session on a turbo/static bike. The Alphamantis system, which a number of testing/coaching companies offer to riders at velodromes, is relatively affordable, especially if two riders share a session. While one is testing, the other is adjusting and tweaking their set-up ready for their next run.

WIND TUNNEL

Despite the unrealistic nature of a wind tunnel, this environment is the ultimate in testing as so many variables can be recorded and controlled, and they can also be manipulated quickly. Over the last few years, wind tunnel testing has become more available and affordable for amateur riders, but it still represents a significant investment.

Train to adapt

Along with off-the-bike work and incrementally working towards a more aggressive position, for time triallists and triathletes the key to adapting to a more aggressive aero position is to train in that position. A lot of long-course triathletes make the mistake of doing the bulk of their long training rides on their road bike, only switching to their triathlon bike towards the end of their preparation. This is a big mistake. If you want to be a successful triathlete or time triallist, you have to put the miles in riding in your race position.

When I was working at British Cycling, Ed Clancy would commute in to the National Cycling Centre from Holmsfirth on his time trial bike just to ensure that his time trial/pursuit position became his default setting. Similarly, if you look at Sir Bradley Wiggins, his position, from pursuit to hour record and longer time trials, barely changes. Because of the time he invested in riding in that position, whether it was for a three-minute team pursuit or a 50km time trial at the back end of a Grand Tour, he could hold that position without undue stress or discomfort.

Off-the-bike work for aero gains

Probably one of the biggest areas you can work on to improve your aerodynamics is your physical ability to attain and hold your position. Simply 'turtling' – rotating your shoulders forward, shrugging them up towards your ears and dropping your head, will have a huge impact on your frontal profile, but achieving and sustaining this takes practice and effort. The routine described on pages 170–175 can have a huge impact on your ability to hold an aerodynamic position.

Time trial and non-drafting triathlon bike fit

Time trial and triathlon bike fit is a balancing act between opening up the hip angle (saddle up) to optimise power and being able to maintain an aerodynamic position (i.e. a flatter back) while still being able to breathe.

Four points you should consider:

▶ The best position is the fastest.
▶ The fastest position works within the constraints of the rider's unique biomechanical profile.
▶ The fastest position must be sustainable for the duration of the rider's chosen event.
▶ If sustainability and aero profile come into conflict, choose sustainability.

▶ Fit window for time trialling

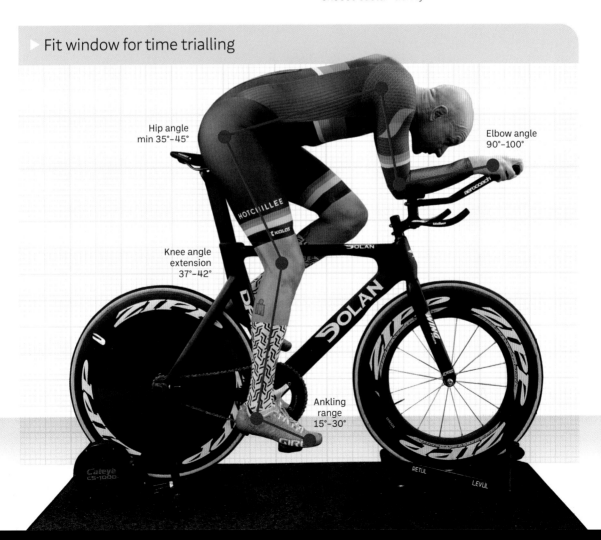

Hip angle
min 35°–45°

Elbow angle
90°–100°

Knee angle
extension
37°–42°

Ankling
range
15°–30°

The last point is the most important.

The increased saddle height and decreased setback rotates the pelvis forward and brings the rider more over the top of the bottom bracket and pedals – a better position from which to generate power.

Due to this, the acceptable level of knee forward of foot changes; the KOPS rule (see page 48) can no longer be applied. The front end – drop and reach – is longer and lower to allow the rider to support his weight through his elbows and adopt a more aero position. This has the effect of lowering the angle of the trunk or back. For most people, adopting an acceptable and sustainable lower frontal position than their road position represents the first gains to be made in this event – you can worry about drag and other factors later on.

So now we have more power and an aerodynamic position. Unfortunately, it is not as straightforward as that.

Can you save your legs for the run?

In triathlon you have to get off your bike and run – a full marathon in the case of an Ironman. Many triathletes and even respected triathlon coaches talk in terms of a bike position 'saving their legs for the run', but from a muscular work and fatigue perspective this just isn't the case. What you can achieve, though, especially by using shorter cranks, is to open up the hip angle on the bike and make the transition from bike to run far smoother. A good analogy is how you feel getting out of a car after a long car journey. If you've been all cramped up in an old Mini, you're going to feel a lot stiffer and sore than if you'd driven a more spacious and luxurious car. Your position on the bike can't save your quads for the run, but it can impact how you feel when you first start running.

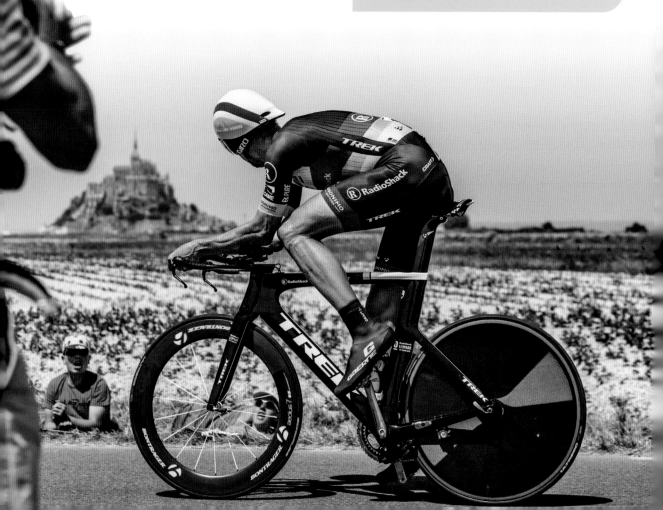

Some possible pitfalls

Because of the lower front end, the hip angle closes more at top dead centre of the pedal stroke than in road cycling, and the chest and diaphragm can become compressed, making it hard to breathe. Sustainability of position is not important solely for maintaining posture and comfort, but also for long-term health. The first of these – the closure of the hip angle – presents a significant health issue to those predisposed to iliac artery kinking (see page 117). When adopting a more closed hip angle in progressing an aero position, be aware of the signs and symptoms of iliac artery kinking and seek appropriate advice and help if they appear. As a safeguard against this I work towards not letting the hip

Crank length

As I explained right at the start of this book, in my experience a massively neglected area of bike fit that can have a huge impact on all areas, including remedying some of the issues associated with – and even improving – an aero position, is crank length. Remember, as a general rule, the lower you can get your front end, the more aerodynamic you'll be. However, as you drop lower, this has the effect of closing your hip angle, which can impact negatively on power production, comfort, ability to breathe and, for triathletes, how you'll feel when you get off the bike and try to run. By switching to shorter cranks, you create more room, allowing for a lower position, but still keeping your hips open.

In the build-up to the Rio Olympics, Sir Bradley Wiggins had been focusing on his hour record attempt and was using 177.5mm cranks. He heard that we'd switched the other guys on the team pursuit squad to shorter 165mm cranks and wanted to do the same. In a very Bradley way, rather than adjusting gradually, he went to 170mm the next day and down to 165mm the day after. What he found was that he was able to drop his front end by 30mm and significantly reduce his drag, but, remember, this is a guy who already had a great position.

▶ Safe and unsafe hip angles

Note how the hip angle – the line of the upper leg (femur) compared to the line of the torso (back) – is so much more acute on the right and less than the 'safe' 45 degrees.

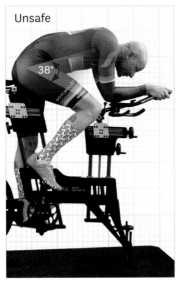

Safe 50°

Unsafe 38°

▶ Compressed breathing

See how the thigh bumps up against the rider's chest due to the closed hip angle caused by the low front end.

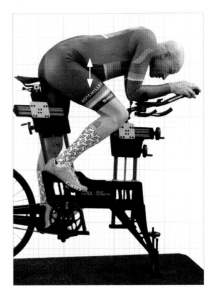

close more than 45 degrees.

For some people, postural and biomechanical limitations mean that in getting a low position they compromise their breathing. Either the ribcage simply cannot expand enough or the diaphragm cannot descend into your tummy or abdomen due to the squashed/compressed nature of the position.

I find a lot of these issues can be avoided if the upper body is supported correctly. On tri-bars, this is solely through the elbows and forearms. Getting the elbow below the shoulder at 90 degrees is a key aim in time trial and triathlon fits – it allows the upper body to relax, minimising energy expenditure. I sometimes look at it like this: it's hard enough trying to breathe effectively when you are cycling flat out, without having to divert 50 per cent of your upper body strength into maintaining a stable position.

The combination of the right stack height under the elbow pads, the right pads to support your elbow and forearms, and correct width is worth spending time over, as is the right bar extension for you to work with.

Contact points

The contact points – saddle and bars particularly – need to be as supportive as can be managed for time trial riding so as to make the position sustainable.

Saddle choice

Probably the key item of kit selection that can make or break a time trial or triathlon position is your saddle. If you're unable to rotate your pelvis, there's no way you'll be able to attain a low front end, a flat back and maintain power production. If your saddle or saddle position is blocking your ability to rotate, or not providing adequate support when you are rotated forward, you're always going to struggle. For triathletes, with far fewer rules restricting their position, getting them rotated forward is far easier. However, if you're riding under UCI rules, especially the one that insists the nose of the saddle has to be 50mm behind the centre of the bottom bracket, it can be trickier. Choosing the right saddle is essential, but also introducing some forward tilt can really help to achieve that forward rotation.

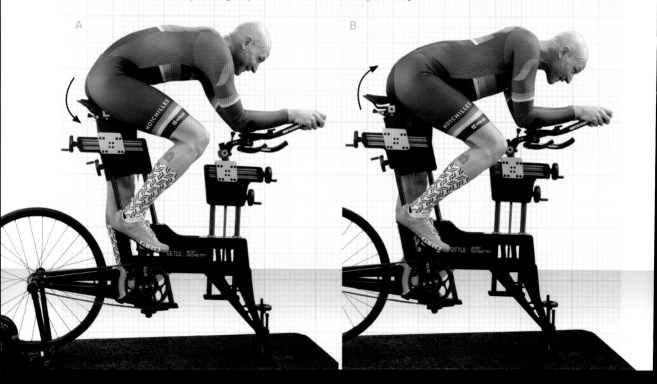

▶ Rotated pelvis in time trial riding

The rider in A has been forced to flex his lumbar and thoracic spine to make the position work, his pelvis being so rotated backwards. The rider in B, by rotating his pelvis forward, flattens his spine nicely.

A

B

In track pursuiting this is exaggerated even more by the increased pressure of the banking that the velodrome creates in the turns. It's no wonder then that exposure to long training bouts of this type of riding often presents us with saddle soreness issues.

Media and viewers often debate whether, when a rider is seen constantly shifting backwards and forward on their saddle in a time trial, this is due to poor position or saddle choice. Both can be responsible, but sometimes it's just a rider creeping forward to optimise their position over the bottom bracket (effectively encroaching on the saddle setback) and shifting back as this becomes uncomfortable to redistribute the load on the undercarriage.

The choice of saddle has to allow the rider to rotate the pelvis forward in the first place. Some people can

▶ Saddle pressure from time trial position

This image graphically shows how little a time trial rider will use of the saddle to bear weight, and how concentrated the saddle pressures can be.

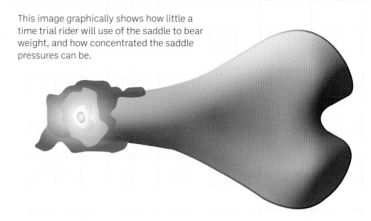

do this on a normal saddle, while others struggle to overcome the constraints of the saddle's shape and hence a whole host of new anatomical saddles have been developed. These are favoured by women, who tend to suffer more from saddle issues in general

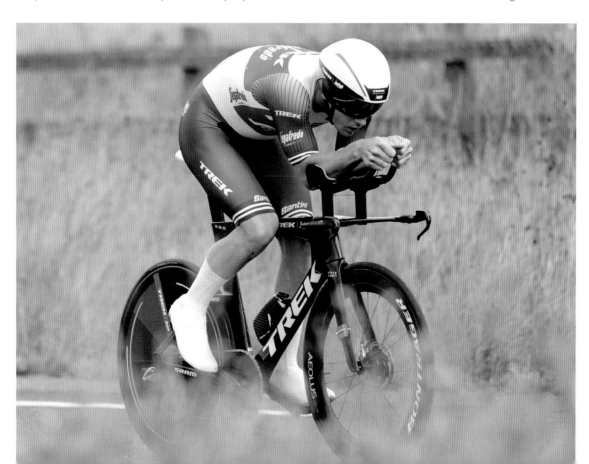

than men. However, I have not found a rationale to explain why some work for certain riders and not for others. My advice is that you have to try different models and see what works for you – some people get on with cutaway saddles, while others find they make the problem worse and prefer a saddle with the best supportive material. If trying out saddles in a shop, remember to rotate forward and shift onto the nose of the saddle as this is where you will more than likely end up in a time trial itself.

Bars

Choice of bars and set-up is important in how the upper body is supported in time trialling because of the increased weight distribution on the arms with the extended reach and drop characteristic of the position, and the fact the rider is rotated forward from the pelvis.

Too much reach and the rider has to use the muscles of the neck and back instead of supporting his or her weight through the forearms and elbow pads – this leads to pain and discomfort and is not sustainable. Too little reach squashes the rider and can lead to difficulty expanding the ribcage/diaphragm and therefore breathing, and can cause back pain as the curvature of the middle back is increased to bring the upper body to the bars.

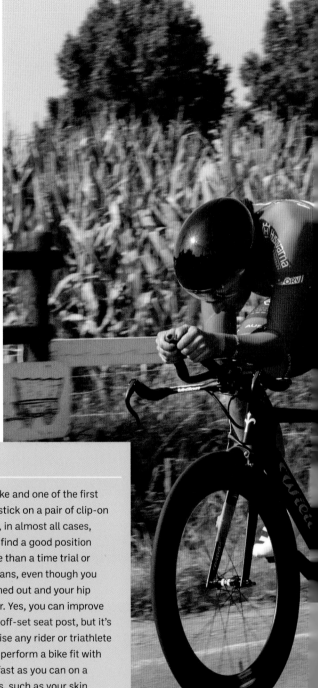

Aero bars on a road bike

Almost all time triallists and triathletes start off on a road bike and one of the first things many do to try and improve their aerodynamics is to stick on a pair of clip-on aero bars. I always say this is like putting lipstick on a pig as, in almost all cases, the geometry of a road bike means it's almost impossible to find a good position with them. Road bikes are significantly longer in the top tube than a time trial or triathlon bike and the seat tube angle isn't so steep. This means, even though you might be able to get your front end lower, you'll be so stretched out and your hip angle so closed down that power output will inevitably suffer. Yes, you can improve things with modifications such as a far shorter stem and an off-set seat post, but it's always going to end up a sub-par compromise. I'd never advise any rider or triathlete to try and fit aero bars on a road bike and certainly wouldn't perform a bike fit with this objective in mind. You'll always be better off getting as fast as you can on a standard road bike set-up, maximising power and easy gains, such as your skin suit and helmet, and then, when you can afford it, investing in a dedicated time trial or triathlon bike.

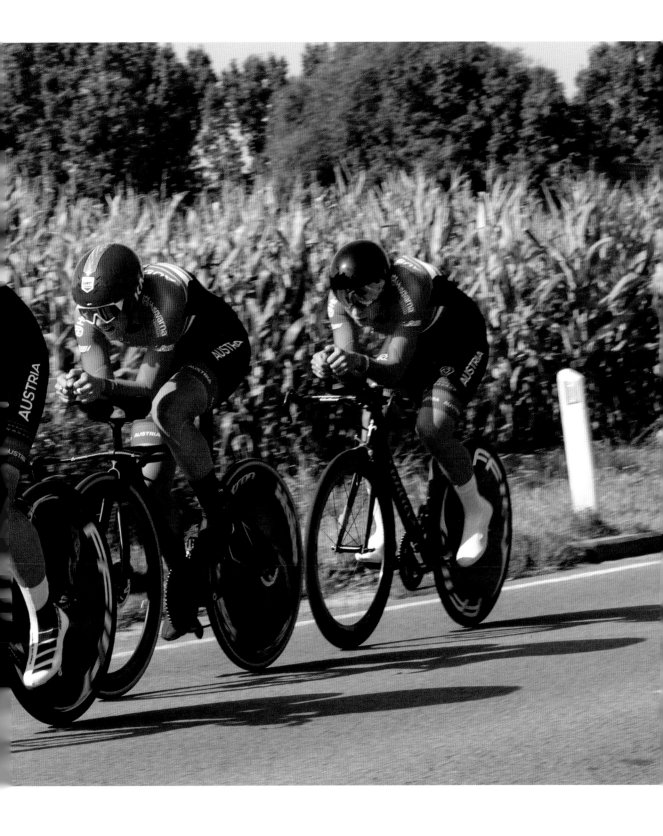

Arm pads

The arm pads on the bars should be positioned on or close to the elbows to allow the rider to effectively bear his or her weight through them. If the arm pads are too far forward this increases the muscular workload needed to stabilise the upper body and leads to fatigue in the arms, shoulders and neck.

The width at which the arm pads are placed is critical and is often overlooked. A very narrow arm position is deemed aerodynamically appropriate, but places a substantial load on the shoulders and upper back musculature. Again, strength and flexibility work off the bike may be necessary to sustain this position.

Wider arm placement where the weight is borne directly below the shoulder joint requires less muscular effort and can allow the rider to drop their head in line with the rest of the torso. However, some riders struggle to control this due to weakness in the muscles between their shoulder blades. Often, they will seek narrower arm pads or bars to prop themselves up and reduce the muscular workload in the middle of the back or shoulders.

UCI rules and regulations

In the first edition of this book I went into the current UCI rules and regulations that were relevant to time trial position and pursuit position on the track in a fair amount of detail, but, within a matter of months, the goal posts had been moved – this included the rule change that I contributed to on saddle angle! So for this edition, if you are competing in a UCI-sanctioned event, you should refer to the current guidelines or, if you're unable or unwilling to wade through them, find a coach or bike fitter who has!

Angling the bars slightly upwards allows the upper body to work less, because it has something to push back against, thus removing the feeling that you are constantly fighting to stop yourself falling off the front of the bike. However, UCI-sanctioned racers should check the constantly changing rules on angles.

▶ Difference in weight distributions for the road and time trial positions

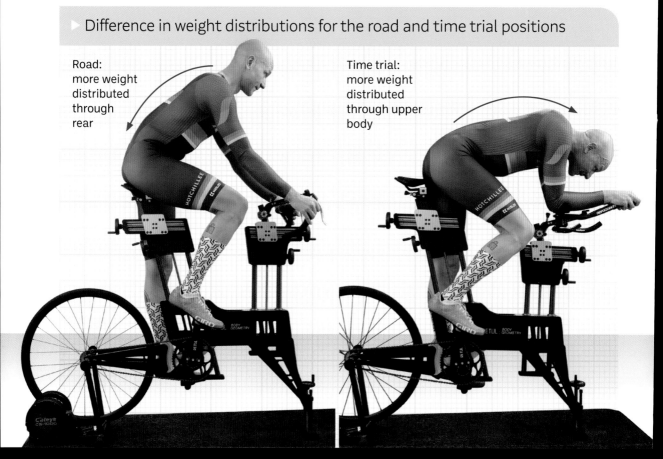

Road: more weight distributed through rear

Time trial: more weight distributed through upper body

▶ Too-long and too-short reach positions

TOO LONG

The elbow angle is way off 90 degrees. The bars are too far away and reach is too long.

TOO SHORT

Note the rider's knee nearly hitting the elbow and bars.

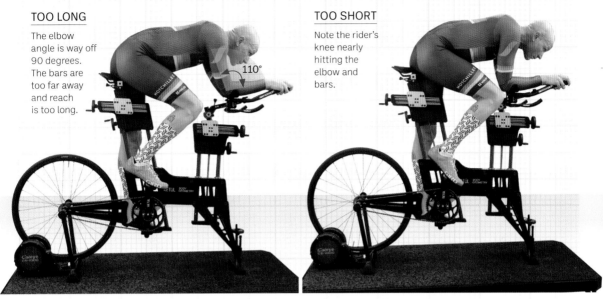

110°

▶ Aero bar width

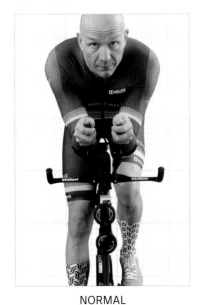

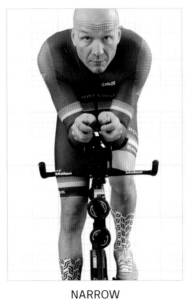

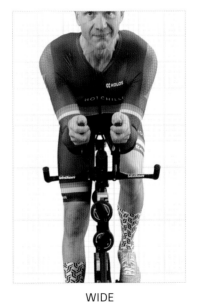

NORMAL

A typical aero bar width.

NARROW

This is more areo – his head drops in nicely. Note the increased tension in the shoulders and upper back though.

WIDE

Some riders will find a wider aero bar postion will allow their head to drop in.

▶ Arm pads too far forward

In A, the rider can support his weight closer to the elbow, reducing the muscular workload that B requires.

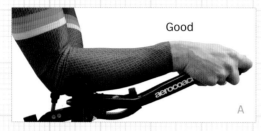

Good

A

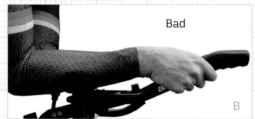

Bad

B

At the end of the upper-limb chain, the hands and wrists should be relaxed and able to move easily. If they are taut and full of tension, work back through the previous points, because this means they are compensating for proximal inaccuracies in the set-up.

A rider's aero position is a reflection of their riding history, flexibility and upper-body strength: to ride an aggressive position with your saddle forward and a low front end, you need good upper-body strength to support your weight, and flexibility to adopt the position, which will test the neck, back, pelvis and hamstrings.

If you don't have the requisite strength, you will soon experience neck pain, a tired upper body (arms, shoulders and back) and tight hips. You need to start your time trial position less aggressively – saddle back, bars up – and start working off the bike on your limitations. If you're serious about getting a good time trial position you may well need to commit to a flexibility and strength programme to get into position and hold yourself there.

▶ Bars angling upwards help a rider to stabilise

In A, the slightly upward orientation of the aero extension gives the rider something to work against and stops the feeling of falling over the front of the bike, and the extra muscular workload involved. In B, the rider looks – and will feel – like he is about to fall off the front of his bike.

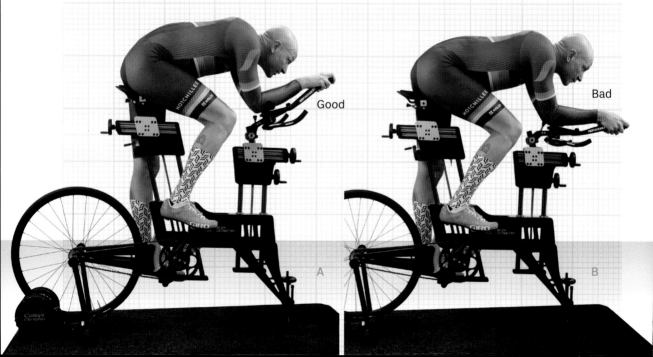

Good

Bad

A

B

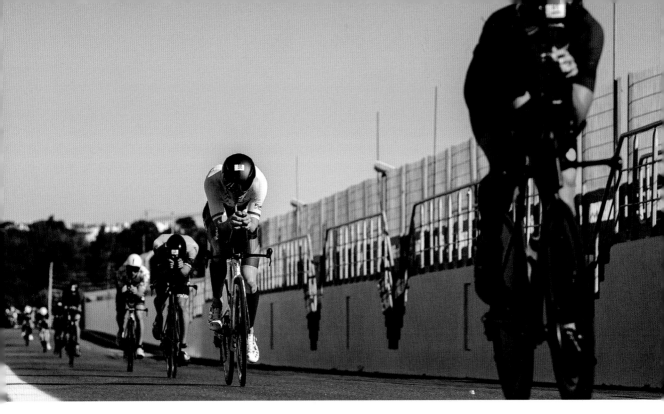

▶ Relaxed hands and wrists

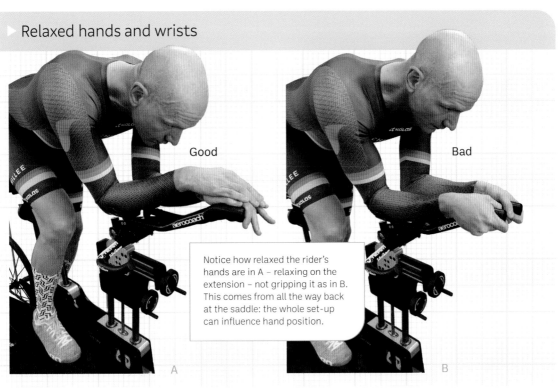

Good

Bad

Notice how relaxed the rider's hands are in A – relaxing on the extension – not gripping it as in B. This comes from all the way back at the saddle: the whole set-up can influence hand position.

A

B

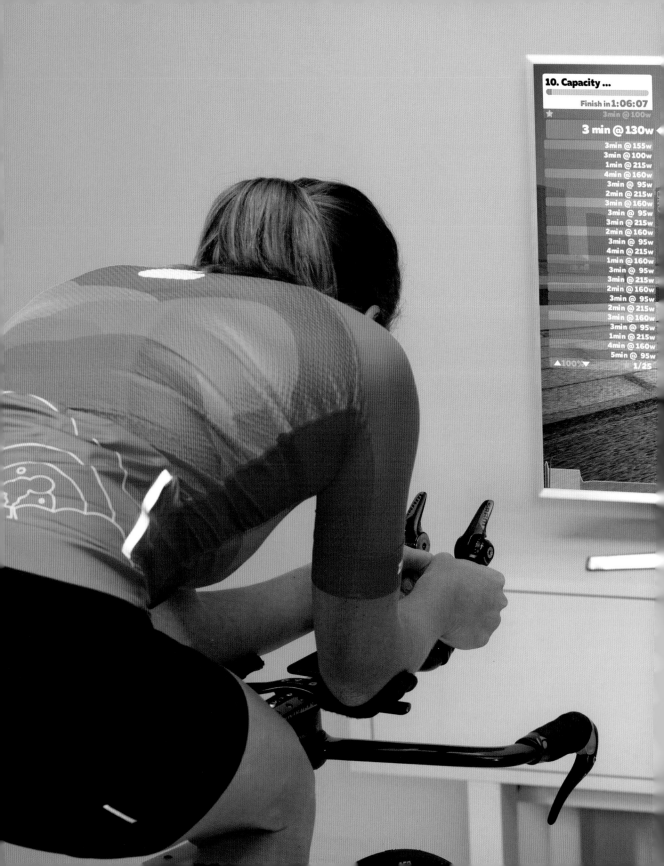

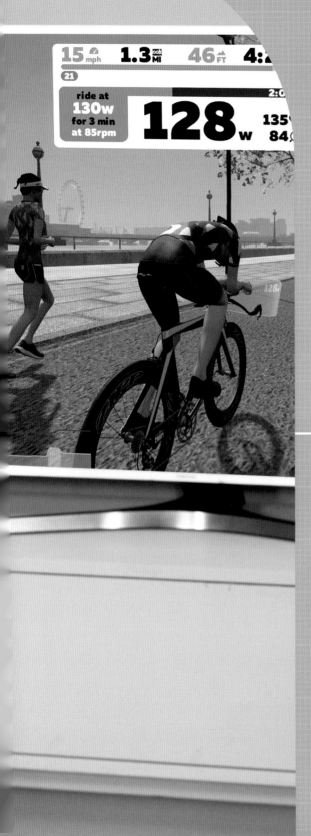

Indoor cycling

Indoor cycling

With modern smart trainers, interactive platforms such as Zwift, and World eRacing championships sanctioned by national governing bodies and the UCI, indoor cycling has transitioned from a necessary winter training evil to a year-round cycling discipline in its own right.

The Covid-19 pandemic also contributed to a massive upswing in participation in indoor cycling and there's a surprisingly large tranche of cyclists who started cycling indoors without any intention or desire to ride outside on roads or trails. There are even a number of elite riders who are now specialising in eRacing and taking home some large prize purses.

During the pandemic, while providing a remote fitting and physiotherapy service, I became increasingly aware of a number of particular issues that indoor cycling can lead to.

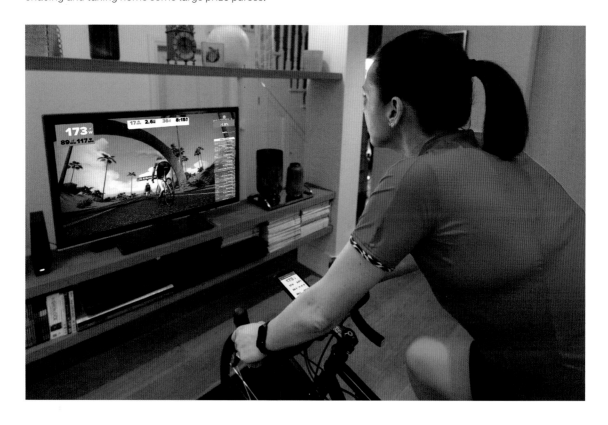

Highlighting any issues

If you have any issues with your position, especially relating to the contact points of saddle, pedals and bars, indoor cycling is going to highlight them and, if ignored, exacerbate them. The simple reason for this is that, unlike when riding outside where you constantly have micro-breaks and positional shifts when you descend, corner, stand to climb a rise and so on, on an indoor trainer you're far more static. Even if your position is perfect, this relentless aspect to indoor riding can mean that you experience discomfort, especially in the saddle region, which you might never have suffered from when riding outside.

▶ A range of indoor trainers

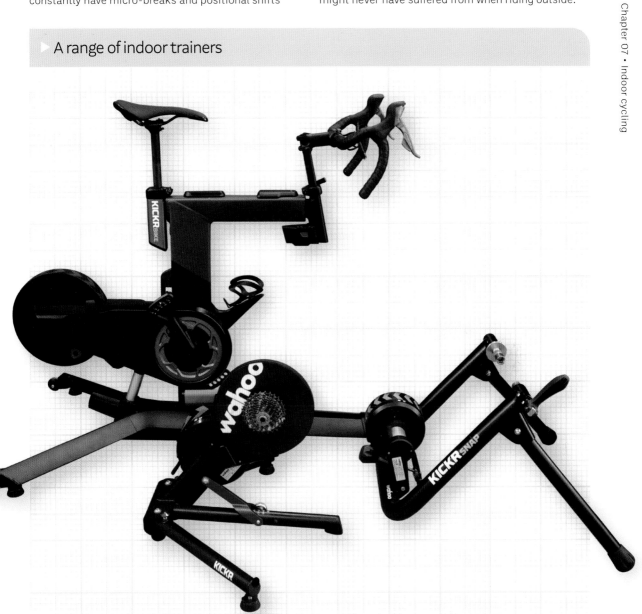

Matching your outdoor riding position

If you're simply dropping your outdoor bike onto a turbo then there won't be any positional changes to consider, but many cyclists have a dedicated bike that they leave set up on the turbo, or have a static bike such as a WattBike, Wahoo Kickr bike or similar. How closely you replicate your outdoor riding position is very dependent on both your indoor and outdoor cycling goals.

Assuming that you're happy with your outdoor position, the number one priority is replicating saddle set-up. This includes the saddle you're using, as many static bikes come fitted with horrendous saddles. Try to dial in saddle height, fore/aft and tilt as close to your road position as you can. Don't forget to check the crank length of your indoor bike as this will impact on your saddle set-up.

If you're using the same shoes and pedals as outside then there shouldn't be any issues here, but if you're using a a pair of dedicated indoor shoes, double-check that cleat positioning is the same.

Once you've ticked these two boxes, if your main goal for indoor cycling is general fitness then you should set up your handlebars to be as comfortable as possible. This probably means having them slightly higher than you would outside.

Similarly, if you're looking to maximise your indoor cycling performance for eRacing, then a less aggressive bar set-up and more upright position than you'd have on the road is the way forward. It will ensure your hips stay open for maximum power production and, by keeping your chest up, will facilitate breathing. There's no benefit in trying to contort yourself into an aero position – it's all about delivering maximum watts to your on-screen avatar!

However, if your indoor cycling is all about improving your performance outdoors, especially for time triallists and triathletes, then taking advantage of indoor sessions to adapt to, and even develop, your position is a no-brainer. In this situation, you should make every effort to replicate your real-life cockpit set-up as closely as possible.

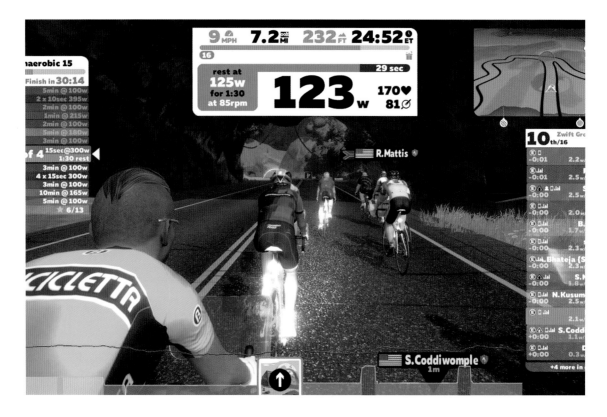

Knee pain

During the lockdown I did notice an increase in riders who, having switched more of their cycling to indoors, were experiencing knee pain. Knee pain on the bike, like any pain, should never be ignored, especially as cycling in general is excellent for knees and often plays a key role in rehabilitation from knee injuries or surgery.

Once I'd drilled down and eliminated any positional issues with these clients, often finding that it was something as simple as saddle positioning or cleat set-up that wasn't quite the same as their outside set-up, I tended to find that there was some slight imbalance or weakness. When riding outside, with the constant shifts in weight distribution and position I've already mentioned, these weren't an issue, but, with the fixed and relentless movement patterns associated with riding indoors, they were compounded and resulted in discomfort. More often than not, some focused release and mobility work sorted the issue.

Anecdotally, a number of riders have also told me that their cadence indoors, especially when trying to sustain high output when eRacing, is significantly lower than it would be riding outdoors. This higher torque pedalling could result in greater stress to your knees, so it's worth bearing in mind.

Foot pain

Indoor cycling means constant pressure through your pedals, so if you suffer from hotspots or foot pain when riding outside, it's likely to be worse when riding indoors. The higher temperatures and lower airflow can also cause your feet to swell, which can further contribute to discomfort. Lighter mesh-style shoes can help improve ventilation and cooling, and try to wear really lightweight, thin socks for both clothing purposes and to give your feet a bit more room. Shoes used for indoor cycling do get soaked through with sweat, so be fastidious about cleaning and drying

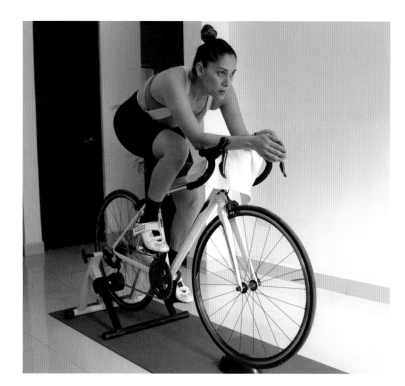

them after sessions or you'll create an ideal breeding ground for bacteria.

Saddle soreness

This is probably the biggest issue that many cyclists have with riding indoors. They can ride outdoors for four or five hours without the slightest hint of saddle soreness, but 30 minutes on an indoor trainer and it's as though they're sat on barbed wire.

The first culprit again is that lack of movement and the simplest remedy for this is to get into the habit of standing up every five minutes or so. Even if it's just for a few seconds, it'll help to relieve pressure and restore blood flow. If you think you're likely to forget, set an alarm on your phone to remind you. Another option is rocker plates, which allow a static bike or bike on a turbo to move slightly underneath you more naturally as you pedal. Some riders swear that these have revolutionised their indoor riding experience, so if soreness is a real issue and you need to spend a lot of time on your indoor trainer, they're definitely worth trying.

The next culprit is the same trinity of heat, moisture and pressure that leads to saddle soreness

Can you learn a perfect pedal stroke?

Some indoor cycling platforms offer real-time pedal stroke analysis and, although this can be interesting and useful in identifying imbalances, I'm sceptical about whether you can use them to develop a smoother and more efficient pedal stroke. You'll often hear cyclists waxing lyrical about *souplesse* and, although there's no doubt that some pros do have wonderfully silky, smooth pedal strokes, they wouldn't have developed this staring at a pedal scan graphic on an indoor trainer. Equally, there are some top cyclists whose pedal stroke is far from smooth, but this doesn't stop them producing big watts for hours on end.

Especially if you're a time-poor amateur cyclist, the time you'd need to invest focusing on pedalling technique to make any sort of lasting change, if indeed you can, simply makes it a gain that's not worth chasing. I know one rider who went down this particular training rabbit hole, spent months doing sessions focused on low-intensity pedalling technique and proudly proclaimed he now had a perfectly even pedal stroke, but he'd shipped about 60W from his FTP. When he then started pushing harder again, his hard-acquired *souplesse* fell to bits and he went straight back to his old pedal pattern.

If your position is correct and you follow a well-designed, structured training plan, your pedal stroke will become more efficient simply with time on the bike. There is some evidence that mountain biking, where you're having to put down power smoothly to maintain traction, and track cycling, where the high cadences on a fixed gear push you through an even pedal stroke, can help with the development of a more even pedal stroke, and, for all round cycling fitness, skills and enjoyment, I'd encourage all riders, especially young ones, to try a range of cycling disciplines.

▶ Increase airflow with a fan

Remember, you can never have too many fans

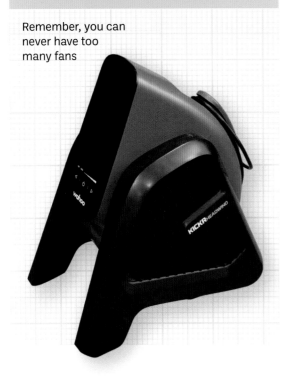

when riding outside. However, when riding indoors, all of these factors are dialled up to 11. It's essential therefore that you follow the steps and advice for preventing saddle soreness on pages 118–126 even more fastidiously.

A lot of riders make the mistake of using old and near-to-the-end-of-their-life shorts for indoor cycling, but out of all the riding you do, the time that you really want well-fitting shorts and pad is when you're on the turbo.

MANAGE YOUR ENVIRONMENT
Having already established the role of heat and moisture in the development of saddle soreness, doing as much as you can to reduce the temperature, increase ventilation and minimise sweating will have a huge impact. You really can't have too many fans or too much ventilation when cycling indoors and, if you're finishing surrounded by a pool of sweat, you haven't got enough. Along with a fan in front of you, there's a lot to be said for having one blowing from behind too. This will increase airflow around your saddle contact area and can have a real impact on soreness.

Think also about how you position any screen you're watching to avoid putting unnecessary strain on your neck. Ideally, you should be looking straight ahead as you would on the road. A bit of consideration to ergonomics can make a big difference to indoor cycling comfort.

PICK YOUR SESSIONS

The ideal sessions to do indoors are high intensity and low duration workouts or races. There's less time for any issues to become a problem and, as you'll be putting a relatively high load through your pedals during hard efforts, there will be less weight on your saddle and therefore less soreness. If possible, for this reason, try to do recovery rides and any endurance work outside.

POST-RIDE ROUTINE

Get out of your sweaty kit, showered and dry straight after your session – checking out your data or where you placed can wait. Bearing in mind what I've already said about indoor riding potentially exacerbating any imbalances or tightness, dedicating some time to flexibility, mobility and release work can be a good idea.

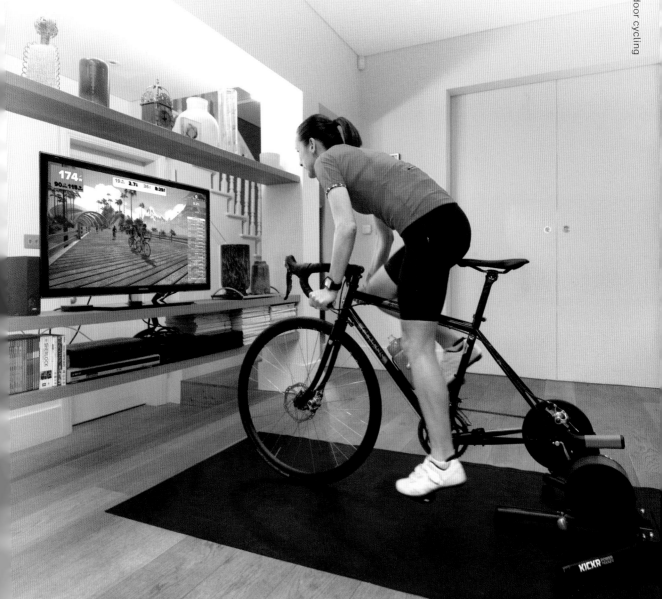

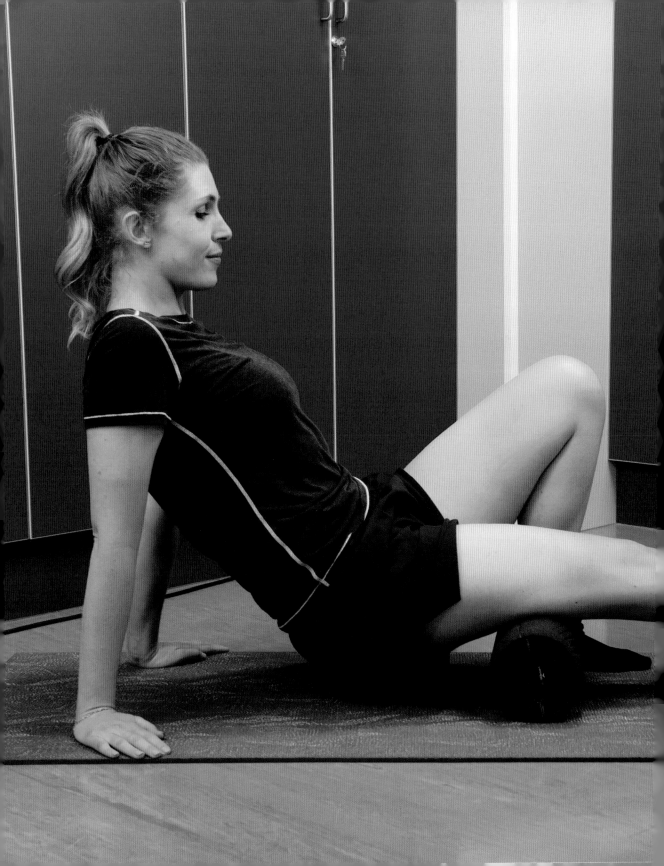

08

Off-the-bike work to help cycling and bike position

Off-the-bike work to help cycling and bike position

So the bike is adjustable and the human adaptable. We have discussed how to adjust the bike and how some of us are just not very adaptable. But there are ways we can influence our bodies to become more adaptable and help them evolve towards accepting that new more aero or more powerful position.

In the same way, though, that every rider's position, training plan and what they like to eat on the bike is different, so too is the off-the-bike work they should be doing. A one-size-fits-all routine that you see in so many cycling training plans is likely to be untargeted, ineffective and potentially dangerous.

This particularly applies to loaded exercises in the gym. Cycling is brilliant for health and fitness in so many ways, but the movement patterns it involves are very limited and linear, and this tends to mean that cyclists often have limited range of movement and poor control through that range. If you try to perform, for example, a barbell squat – a staple of many 'cycling strength routines' – with these limitations, good, safe and effective form is practically impossible. This doesn't just apply to amateur riders either. When I was working with British Cycling there were plenty of riders on the endurance squads who I wouldn't let anywhere near a squat rack!

Having written the first edition of this book, and thinking about this issue more and more, I realised that the subject of off-the-bike conditioning for cyclists needed a whole book dedicated to the subject. This led me, in collaboration with Martin Evans, former Senior Strength and Conditioning Coach at the English Institute of Sport (EIS) and Lead Strength and Conditioning Coach for British Cycling, to write *Strength and Conditioning for Cyclists: Off the Bike Conditioning for Performance and Life*.

I really do view that book as a companion book to this one and would strongly recommend, if you're wanting to incorporate off-the-bike conditioning into your training routine, which I'd argue all cyclists should,

that you refer to it. It's based around a simple and easy-to-perform DIY functional movement screening that is similar to the one we used when assessing riders on the Great Britain Cycling Team. This assessment will pinpoint your limitations and allow you to create a targeted, personalised and progressive off-the-bike conditioning programme. It starts off taking you through corrective exercises to improve your mobility, moves on to developing control and strength through that improved range, and finally progresses to adding load to the movements.

Why do off the bike work?

One of the fundamental principles of training is specificity. This simply states that the best training for a given activity is performing that activity. So the best training for cycling is, unsurprisingly, getting out and turning those pedals over. It may seem contradictory therefore, especially if the time that you can devote to training is limited, to suggest that you devote some of it to off-the-bike training.

Until very recently, the mindset that the only worthwhile training for cycling is cycling prevailed within the sport and, even now, within less progressive professional teams, the benefit of off-the-bike training is viewed with scepticism. Not so long ago the only 'cross training' that riders would do might be some cross-country skiing at the off-season get-together training camp. The change in mindset to embrace off-the-bike training was a real seismic shift in the sport that I was lucky enough to be part of during my time at British Cycling.

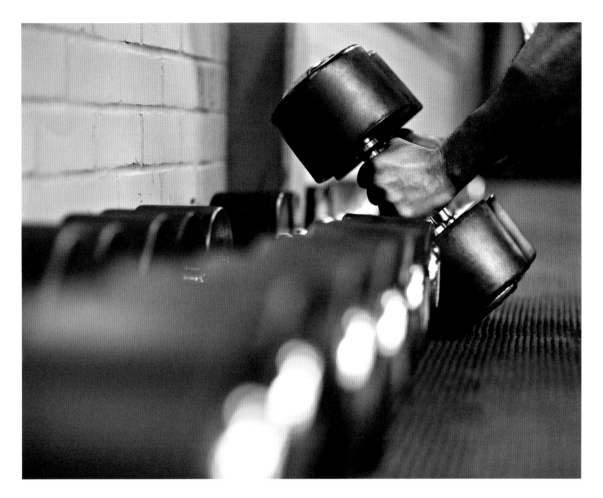

Strength training had been an accepted component of track sprinters' training for years. In fact, they're often jokingly referred to as weightlifters who occasionally ride bikes. With certain track endurance disciplines, specifically the team pursuit, evolving to demand more sprint-type performances, the coaches started to prescribe more gym work for the endurance riders. The results were good and the riders started to notice improvements in others areas of their riding too, including on the road. The riders and coaches took this knowledge to their pro road teams and slowly it became an accepted part of the training routine for most road cyclists.

Off-the-bike training, if done correctly, can be directly beneficial to your cycling. It can improve your peak power production and make you more stable and efficient when pedalling. It can help you to hold a more aerodynamic position and generally be more comfortable on the bike.

Almost more important, though, are the indirect benefits. As I've already said, cycling works your body in very limited and fixed patterns. This means that, although you can be incredibly strong on the bike, if you're challenged outside those confines you expose yourself to injury risk. Whether it's gardening, lifting the shopping out of the car or some DIY, a loading pattern that you're not used to can easily cause injury and result in time off the bike. Additionally, the biomechanical issues that arise from the amount of time we spend seated in modern life, whether working at a desk or driving, for example, are compounded by the hunched over flexed position that cycling involves. The resulting tight hip flexors, stiff lower back and poorly functioning glutes can manifest in a number of problems, both on and off the bike.

What to do now

Although I'd strongly urge you to get and start using the book I wrote with Martin, there are a number of exercises that are of benefit to all cyclists. Mobility work can be used to correct the tightness and imbalances associated with both cycling and a largely seated lifestyle. These exercises will also be beneficial in that they will allow you to hold a better position on the bike. This aspect is particularly relevant to cyclists who are targeting a more aggressive or aerodynamic position, such as time triallists and triathletes.

This sequence of exercises is targeted, focused and, in terms of time invested, will deliver good bang-for-your-buck gains. Consistency is key to off-the-bike conditioning and, if you're presented with a huge list of exercises that take hours to do, I know that it's just not going to happen. We're all pressed for time and, even when working with full-time riders, I've seen that it's pointless prescribing long multi-exercise routines. I remember Bradley Wiggins coming to me with a list of 27 exercises that his

The common misconception about stretching that I'm keen to dismiss is that it lengthens muscles. This is simply untrue as, with fixed points of origin and insertion, muscle length is essentially fixed. No amount of acute or short-term stretching will lengthen muscles and the only time that muscles do lengthen is when you're growing or under years – and I mean years – of sustained stretch loading. What stretching does is to address muscles' heightened sensitivity to ranges of movement beyond those which you experience when sitting on your bike or at your desk. This perceived tightness, if left unaddressed, can easily lead to imbalances, poor muscle function and potentially pain or injury.

then team had given to him – he was wondering when he'd fit in actually riding his bike! A short routine of effective and targeted exercises done well and regularly are far better than an epic routine done haphazardly every so often.

▶ Foam rollers and trigger point balls

Mobility

Mobility work draws on tool-assisted self manual therapy (TASMT) – using a foam roller or trigger ball to release an area, and then stretching, to work it through an extended range of motion. Almost all cyclists would benefit from focused mobility work throughout the year, as it helps to address imbalances and tightness both from cycling and from daily life. As I've said, it can also improve your position and comfort on the bike, and increase your resilience to injury from movements and activities outside cycling.

HOW OFTEN?

The routine suggested starting on page 170 takes just over 30 minutes to complete and covers most of the classic areas where both cycling and desk time can cause problems.

The more you can do of this type of work the better really, but at the minimum you should aim to do two to three focused bouts each week. You will probably find certain pairs of exercises feel tougher and that may indicate an area that needs working on. There's no reason why you can't work on certain movements daily or even multiple times per day.

When?

The advice that used to be given for traditional stretching routines was to do them immediately post-exercise. However, the last thing you want to do when you come in cold and wet from a long hard ride or dripping with sweat from a gruelling session on the turbo is roll around on a mat. It's uncomfortable and you're unlikely to do a decent job. You're better off getting clean, warm and fed, and then dedicating some quality time to mobility work. In fact, you can work on this routine at any time, even in front of the television in the evening.

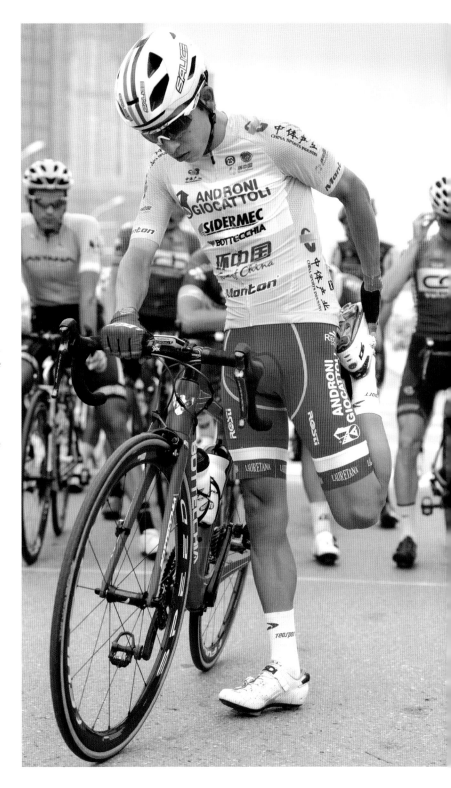

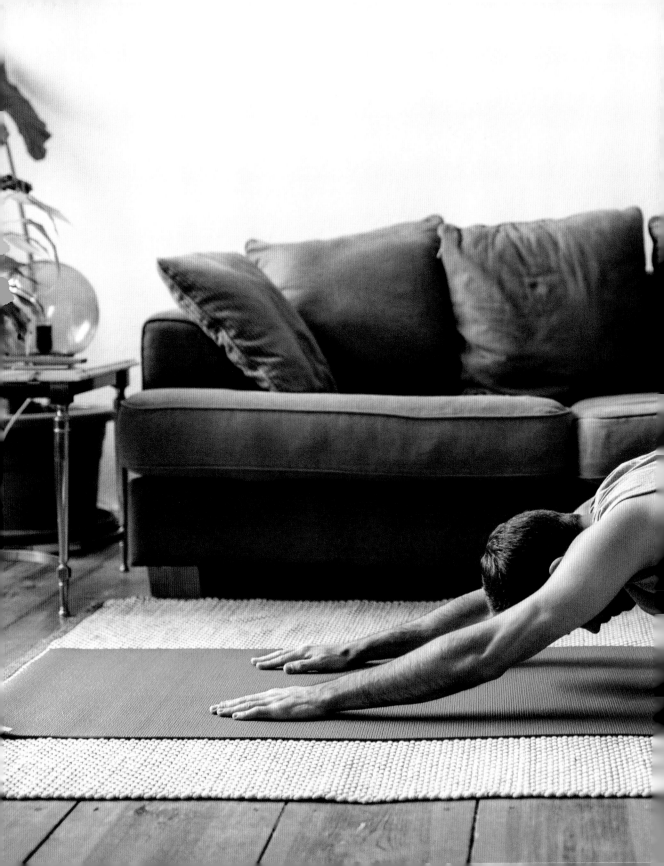

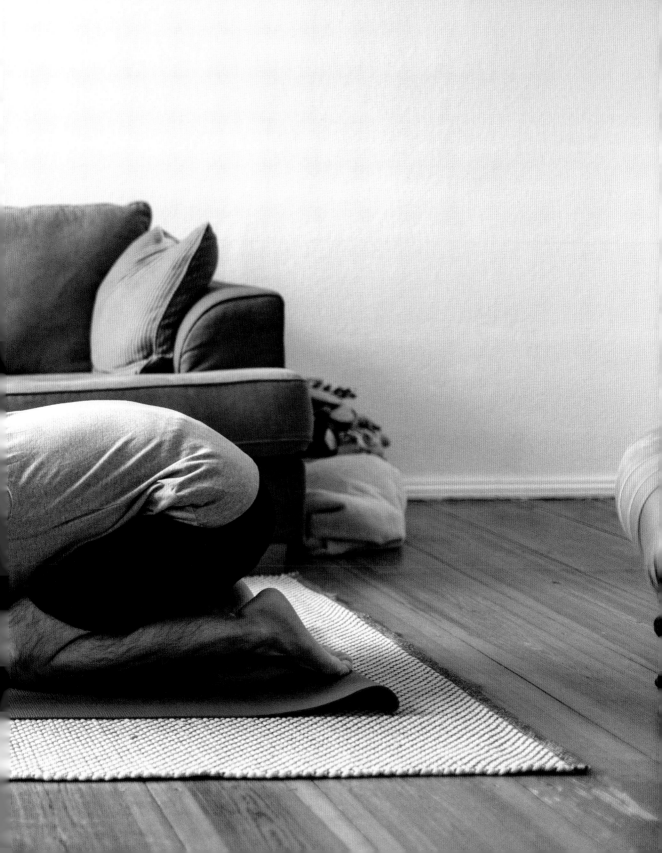

Mobility routine

The A exercise is always tool-assisted self manual therapy (TASMT).

▶ Whether using the foam roller or trigger point ball, don't just roll backwards and forward. Explore the area you're working on, shift your body weight around to change the emphasis and, when you find tight spots, oscillate over them until they release.
▶ Spend at least 2 minutes on each area or side before moving on.
▶ Never roll over bone.
▶ Many people, especially women, experience bruising when first starting foam rolling. This is common, but seek advice if you're worried by it.
▶ If you experience any unusual pain or sensations, consult with a qualified medical professional.

The B exercise is always a stretching movement.

▶ Move and develop the stretch, don't just hold it passively.
▶ Once you find the limit of your movement or a tight area, breathe deeply and try to work through it.
▶ Avoid bouncing or trying to force the stretch.
▶ Hold and develop each stretch for 30-90 seconds.

1a Quad smash with foam roller

Cycling demands a lot of work from your quads, but it's equally the time we spend seated at our desks and driving that contributes most significantly to problems with these muscle groups.

▶ Adopt a plank position over the foam roller with your body weight supported by your elbows, forearms and toes.
▶ With the roller positioned mid-thigh, lower yourself so that the majority of your weight is on the roller.
▶ Rotate to one side to focus your weight on the leg you want to work on.

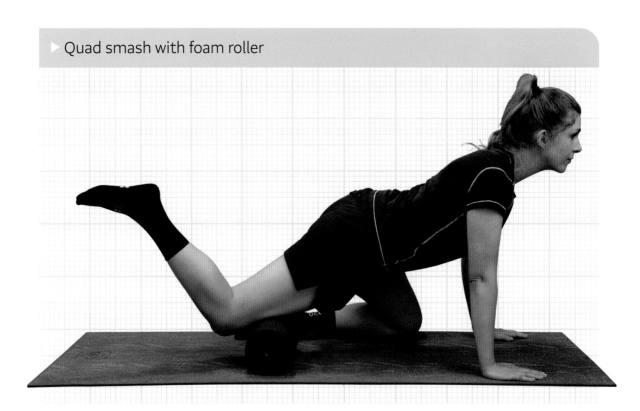

▶ Quad smash with foam roller

- Bend the knee of the working leg and, by slowly rolling back and forth, and rotating your body further to cover the outside areas of your thigh, seek out tight spots.
- When you find a spot, oscillate on and off it for 30–45 seconds, or until you feel it release.
- Find another tight spot and repeat this process, covering the whole thigh before moving on to your other leg.
- You'll typically find you need to focus more on the outside of the muscle.

1b Bulgarian squat

You probably spend a vast proportion of your time sitting at a desk or driving your car, which is then compounded by the hours you spend on your bike.

All this time spent in a leaning forward seated position leads to tight hip flexors, which can be responsible for discomfort both on and off the bike. This dynamic squat is an excellent way to counter tight hip flexors.

- Elevate your rear foot on a bed or bench.
- Squeeze your glutes – you might find this is enough to begin to initiate a stretch.
- Keeping your glutes tight, bend the front knee until you feel a deep stretch through your hip flexors.
- Hold for 30–90 seconds, three times on each side.

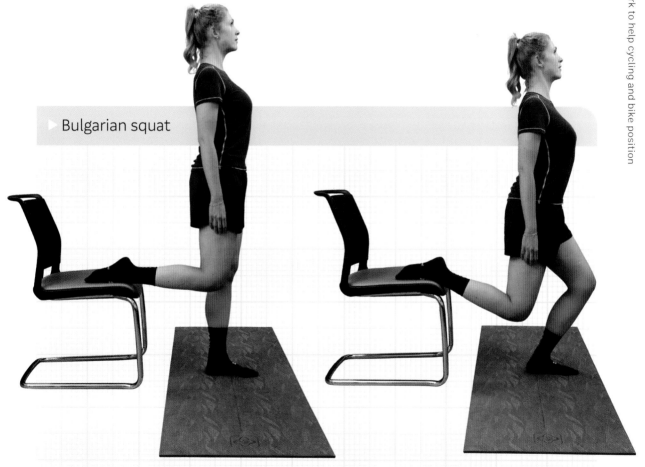

▶ Bulgarian squat

2a Glute smash with foam roller

The glutes muscle group composes the whole of your buttocks and is one of the most powerful in the body. They generate power and thrust in most movements, including running and cycling, by extending the hip. If restricted in their range, you'll be missing out on some of this power and your ability to rotate your pelvis on the hip will be limited. This could also prevent you from achieving an aerodynamic riding position.

► Sit on the foam roller with your legs bent and your hands directly below your shoulders.
► Rotate onto the buttock that you want to work on and, to intensify the movement, cross the leg of the opposite side over your thigh.
► Roll back and forth, changing the amount you rotate your body, to explore the whole buttock for areas of tightness or restriction.
► If you find a tight spot, oscillate on and off it for 30–45 seconds or until you feel it release.
► Repeat for the other buttock.
► You can use a trigger point ball for a more intense and focused version of this exercise.

2b Glute stretch

A great stretch for the glutes and a perfect one for doing in front of the TV.

► Kneel on all fours and then bring your left leg through, placing it flat on the floor with a 90-degree bend at the knee and parallel to your pelvis.
► Extend your right leg out behind you, rotating your knee under so that your knee and toes are on the floor.
► Sit back into the stretch, aiming for a straight and level pelvis. Your belly button should be in line with the inside of your left thigh.
► Lift your chest up and breathe through the stretch.
► Experiment with dropping your chest down towards the floor and adding more rotation. Gently work back and forth through any restrictions.
► Change sides and work on the other glute.
► If you struggle to get your hips straight, place a block under your hip, as shown in the illustration.

► Glute smash with foam roller

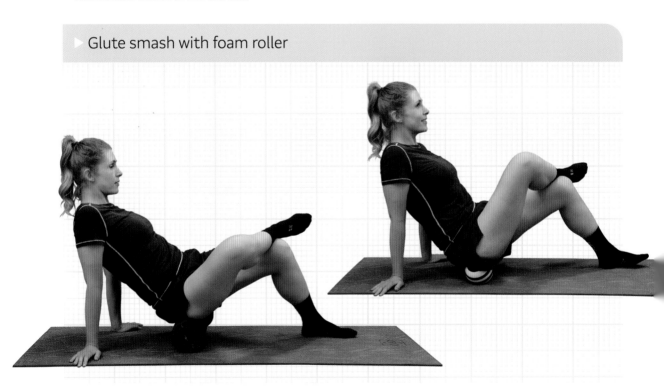

3a Hamstring smash with foam roller

Cyclists often present with tight or restricted hamstrings, because cycling is a closed activity where you are locked in a fixed movement pattern and the knee doesn't typically extend beyond 35 degrees at the bottom of the pedal stroke. As we've already discussed, if a muscle isn't regularly taken through its full range, in the case of the hamstring a fully straightened leg, it will become restricted. As well as creating possible problems off the bike when full extension of the leg is required, tight hamstrings can also affect your riding negatively. Tight hamstrings can be a contributing factor to lower back pain and, as they limit your ability to rotate your pelvis forward, can force you to flex entirely from your lower back and spine. This can compromise your ability to attain and hold an aerodynamic position, which is of particular relevance to time triallists and triathletes.

▶ Glute stretch

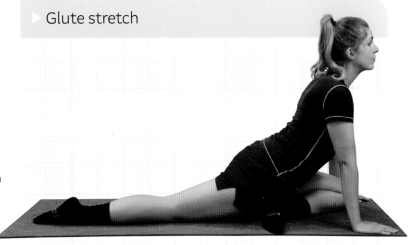

▶ Hamstring smash with foam roller

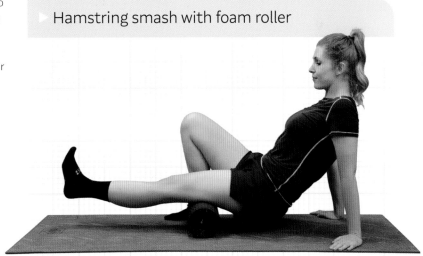

▶ Start in a seated position with your hands directly under your shoulders and the roller positioned under the backs of your knees.

▶ Bend the knee of the leg you're not working on and shift the majority of your body weight onto the leg still on the roller.

▶ Roll back and forth to mid-thigh and look for areas of tightness. Rotate your foot outwards to focus on your outer thigh and inwards to concentrate on the inner.

▶ If you find a tight spot, oscillate on and off it for 30–45 seconds, or until you feel it release.

▶ Shift your start position so that the roller is now positioned mid-thigh. Repeat the process above, but now working on the top half of your hamstrings up to your buttocks.

▶ Repeat the whole process on your other leg.

▶ You'll typically find you need to focus more on the outside of the muscle.

3b Posterior thigh opener

There are a huge variety of hamstring stretches, but this is one of the most effective. Again, don't just hold a static stretch, this is an active exercise. Bend and straighten your leg to apply and release load.

▶ Lie on your back and loop a strap around your left foot.
▶ Bring your knee towards your chest.
▶ Apply tension to your hamstring by straightening your knee. Increase the intensity by bending and straightening your leg.
▶ Repeat with the other leg.

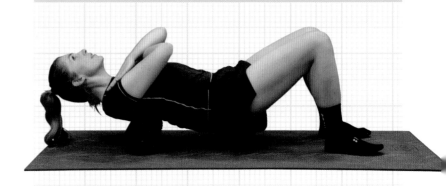

▶ Thoracic spine extension smash

4a Thoracic spine extension smash

This exercise focuses on creating more optimal thoracic extension, which is essential for holding an aerodynamic position. Extending over a foam roller, or a peanut if the large roller is too difficult, also gives a great release feeling after a long day on the bike or behind a desk.

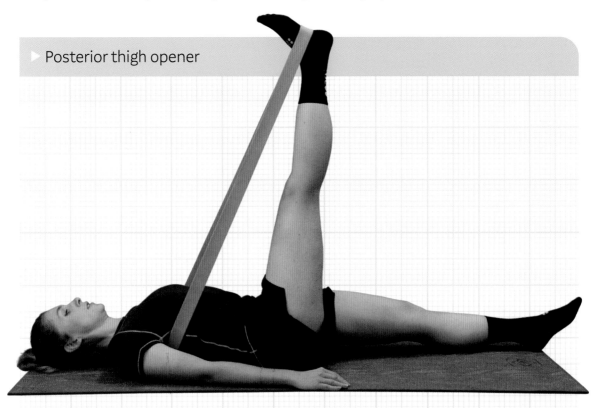

▶ Posterior thigh opener

- Adopt a position as if you were about to perform sit-ups and position the foam roller or peanut so that it's at the base of your ribcage.
- Wrap your arms around yourself and actively pull your shoulders forward.
- Extend over the roller by arching your back.
- Spend time in this position until you feel change.
- Come out of extension, keeping your arms wrapped around you, as if you're doing a sit-up. Allow your backside to move towards your feet, shifting the position of the roller further up your back.
- Extend back over the roller and keep working in this way all the way up to the base of your neck.
- Increase the extension and intensity by squeezing your glutes and pushing your hips up.

4b Recumbent kneeling lat stretch

As the lats are such large muscles, restrictions in them can have negative impacts both on and off the bike. Affecting both shoulder mobility and also the spine, they are a key muscle group for good form in a huge number of common gym exercises, as well as achieving a good aerodynamic position on the bike.

- Kneel and reach forward with your hands, placing them on the mat in front of you about shoulder-width apart.
- Keeping one hand where it is, place the other hand on top of it.
- Sit back gently towards your heels, making sure your hands stay in position.
- You should feel a stretch develop as you move backwards and, due to the hand position, should feel it on one side more than the other.
- Repeat with your hand position reversed.
- You can advance the stretch by side-bending away from the lower hand side or by elevating your hands on a bench or Swiss ball.

▶ Recumbent kneeling lat stretch

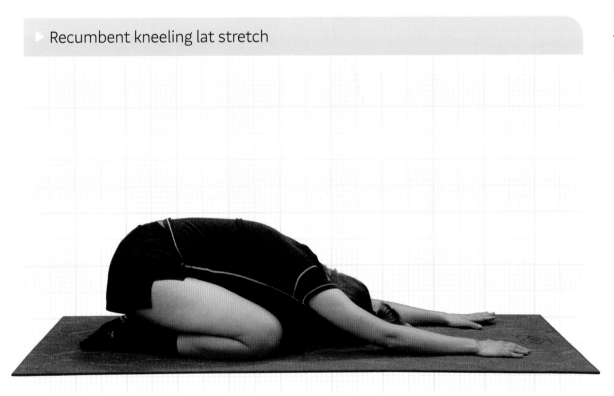

Busting the core myth

For many years you haven't been able to read a fitness magazine without coming across an article extolling the importance of core strength and core stability. Even in cycling-specific publications, stability ball work and other core-focused exercises have been touted as universally beneficial for preventing back pain and improving cycling performance.

I believe that we need to clear away the hype surrounding the core and reassess its role and importance to cycling.

Where it all came from

In the 1990s, research in Australia suggested that weakness in one small muscle of the body's trunk, the transverse abdominus (TrA), was responsible for the majority of lower back pain. With back pain such a prevalent complaint in modern society, the physiotherapy world jumped on this universal cure-all, the fitness industry followed and the core stability craze began. Small, precise and isolated movements that targeted the TrA were not only being prescribed for people suffering from back injuries, but for fitness enthusiasts and athletes searching for performance gains and injury prevention.

The problem

One of the biggest issues with isolating the TrA is that it doesn't actually work in isolation. It works with every other muscle that makes up the abdominal wall in multiple roles, of which spinal stabilisation is only one. Follow-up research has failed to show any conclusive link between back pain and weakness of the TrA in isolation. Even when patients have recovered from bad backs after performing TrA-focused rehabilitation, it's not clear whether the exercises were responsible. They might have improved anyway due to rest and avoiding performing the activities that were aggravating their backs.

There's also the placebo effect to consider.

The benefits of these extremely narrowly focused, reductionist and often lying-down exercises to sports performance are even less clear. They have their place in a rehabilitation scenario, but in other sporting contexts have been mis-sold. Knowing how to prescribe and progress them requires in-depth knowledge and an extremely intensive approach. For the vast majority

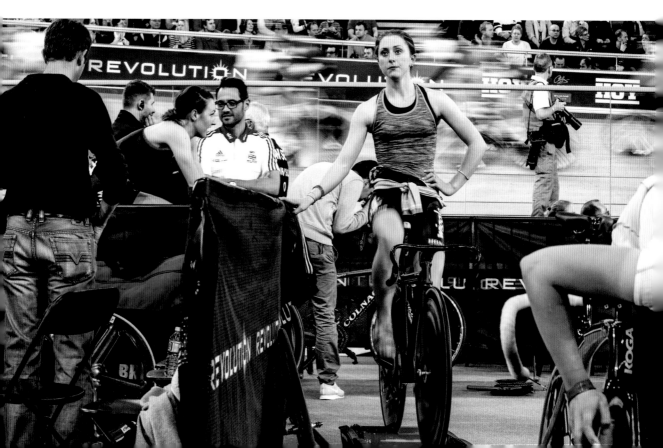

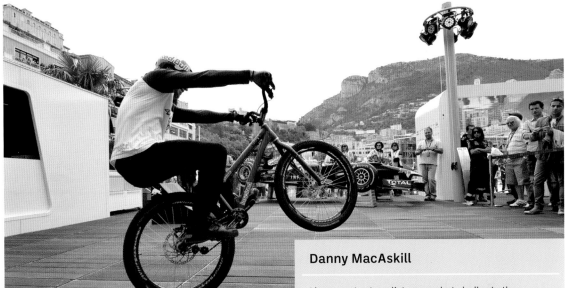

of time-starved cyclists, who already have reasonable functional fitness for cycling and life in general, time spent on these types of exercises without detailed instruction is often time wasted.

Apples have cores, cyclists don't

During my time at British Cycling, the phrase 'core stability' was phased out and instead 'functional trunk strength' and 'robustness' were the watchwords. Functional trunk strength and coordination is what is needed to be able to pedal strongly and perform on-the-bike tasks such as putting on a rain cape. Robustness is the capacity to absorb training and avoid injury both on and off the bike.

If you imagine performance as being a pyramid, cycling-specific fitness is the point at the very top. Relevant strength work might not directly benefit your performance on the bike, but it will indirectly – by building a wider base of robustness and conditioning to your pyramid. This in turn will allow your point to rise higher through an improved ability to cope with consistent training and avoiding lay-offs due to injury.

What does this mean for me?

As a sportive rider, aspiring racer or seasoned club run regular, you're probably already able to ride your bike

Danny MacAskill

I know a stunt cyclist somewhat similar to the famous Danny MacAskill. He once visited a physiotherapist complaining of back pain. He was told he had a poor core and needed to do some simple remedial exercise for it to resolve. This is where my profession lets itself down. So blind has it become – with the whole 'core fixes everything' mantra – that we miss the relevant points too often. I doubt anyone who has seen what Danny MacAskill can do on a bike would dare argue that he lacks core control. The stunt rider I know basically had a sore back from landing constantly on it while perfecting his bike-jumping skills – nothing to do with poor core strength!

for multiple hours and perform the day-to-day tasks and movements that your non-cycling life involves. If this is the case, then the exercises that are typically prescribed for 'core strengthening' will have little relevance or benefit to you. Even if you do sometimes suffer from a sore back on the bike, this can be inevitable after a few tough hours in the saddle, and could be down to your position on the bike or due to factors completely unrelated to cycling. If back pain is limiting you either on or off the bike, refer to the relevant section in this book (see pages 126–129) and, if necessary, consult with an appropriately qualified professional. Devoting your valuable time to exercises that are not proven to help with either back problems or cycling performance is pointless.

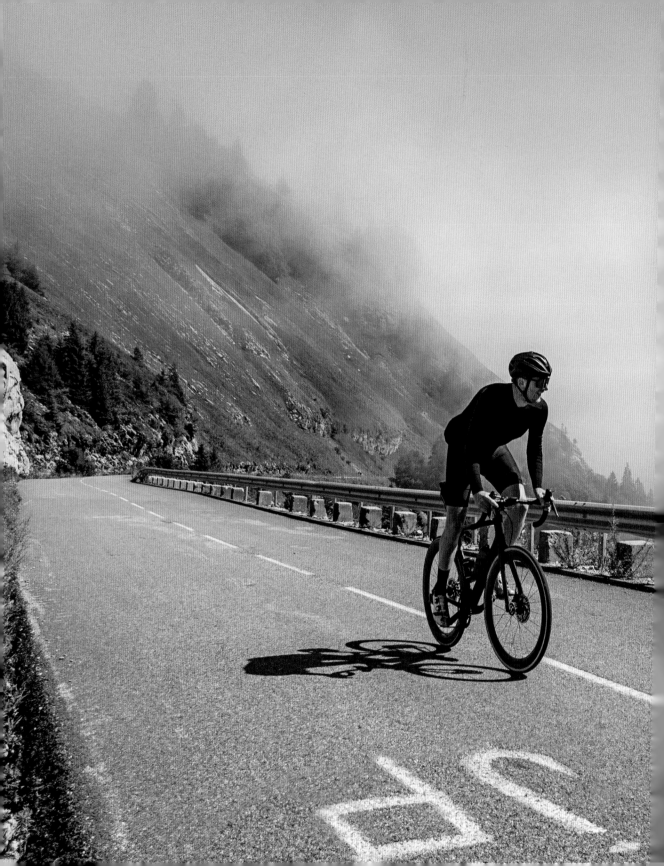

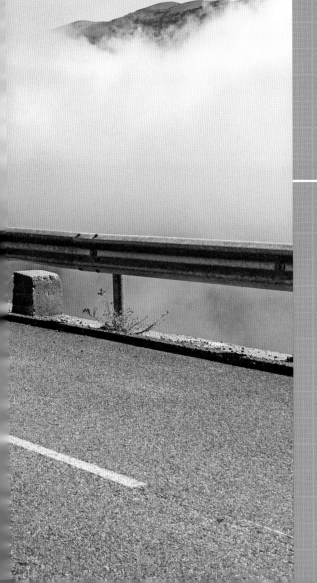

09

Case studies

Case studies

It can sometimes be hard to put together the pieces of your own particular puzzle – be it a bike position issue or a medical problem. I find a useful method of conveying information while lecturing is through storytelling. These case studies should serve as a handy opportunity to pick apart a particular situation – recognising ourselves within a case study often gives that Eureka moment.

Case study 1

A 41-year-old office worker has recently taken up cycling and has become an avid fan. However, the longer he rides, the more numb his hands become. He's also noticed his triceps become tired as it is hard for him to avoid having his elbows locked out all the time. Lastly, his neck aches towards the end of a longer ride, and afterwards.

He almost certainly has a position with too much drop, forcing him to bear too much weight through his hands, which respond by going numb as the nerves are compressed. The tricep fatigue and locked elbows confirm this, as it's the only arm position able to cope with all the extra weight on the front end. The low front end also means he has to extend his neck a lot more to look up the road, causing strain to the musculature around it.

Solution: Address the excessive drop to the handlebars and redistribute weight away from front end.

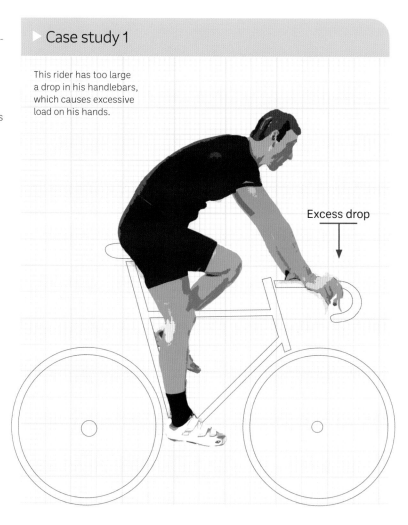

▶ Case study 1

This rider has too large a drop in his handlebars, which causes excessive load on his hands.

Excess drop

Case study 2

A 25-year-old has been riding for some time. He recently had to change saddle. Ever since, he has been feeling numbness in his undercarriage (or genital area), constant lower back pain and suddenly feels like he's now reaching too far forward for the handlebars most of the time. Moving the saddle up and down resolves nothing.

The most likely cause is that the new saddle has not been levelled correctly and is tilted up at the nose. This has the effect of increasing the pressure on the rider's undercarriage and creating numbness. The saddle's rear tilt forces the pelvis to rock backwards, forcing the lower back into much more flexion than it wants to tolerate – hence the lower back pain. He feels like he is reaching to the bars, because despite no positional change his whole body is starting from a much more rearward base of support – the pelvis.

Solution: Level the saddle or even have the nose slightly down (up to -9.0 degrees is considered legal by UCI).

Case study 3

A 24-year-old female rider has been riding for years, quietly suffering from constant saddle soreness on one side. She has noticed that one knee tracks like a piston up and down, but the other tracks in and out in a much more pear-shaped fashion. The foot on this side also seems to point (plantar flex) more at BDC.

These four symptoms combined make me highly suspicious of an actual or functional leg length difference (see pages 129–131). The body has adapted to the asymmetry by laterally moving the pelvis to the short-leg side, thus enabling the shorter leg to reach the pedals, making the short-leg side saddle sore. It also points the foot to help reach the pedal. The shorter leg tracks directly up and down as this is the most direct route. The longer leg has a circular tracking as it has more limb to move through the same space, because the saddle height has been set for the shorter leg.

Solution: Build up the shorter leg with a shim or insole to correct for LLD (see page 131 for more details).

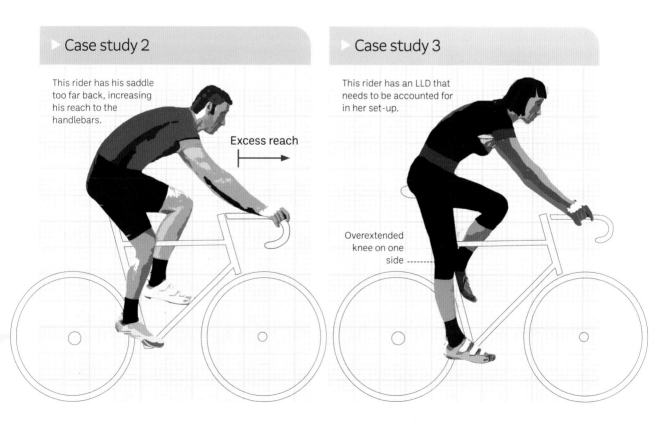

▶ Case study 2

This rider has his saddle too far back, increasing his reach to the handlebars.

Excess reach

▶ Case study 3

This rider has an LLD that needs to be accounted for in her set-up.

Overextended knee on one side

Case study 4

A 30-year-old man recently changed bike. He used exactly the same set-up as on his old bike, but now has to constantly concentrate to stop his heels from hitting the chainstays of the bike, and as a consequence he's developed ITB tightness and some knee pain.

Most likely he has a heels-in, toe-out (duck-footed) walking style. The change in bike has accentuated this as the chainstays are more flared out on his new model and therefore catch his heel on the return stroke of the pedal. To stop this, the lateral structures of the thigh (the VL, or vastus lateralis, and the ITB) are over-activated and start to fatigue/tighten, thus indirectly abnormally loading the patello-femoral joint, causing pain.

Solution: Change to a bike with less flared chainstays or keep the existing bike but use spacers or longer pedal spindles to increase stance width.

Case study 5

A 28-year-old man has seriously taken up time trial riding, converting from the road scene. He has noticed a numb undercarriage, his hips rocking from side to side, ITB/VL tightness and trigger points that will not settle when using his foam roller.

Time trial positioning involves a much higher saddle height. This rider may have started with one that is too high – the pelvis ideally rocks forward in time trialling, but with too high a saddle its motion is blocked, causing the numbness underneath. The rocking of the hips is down to the legs trying to reach the pedals in an effective manner. The overreaching of the knee joint causes the ITB to become irritated.

Solution: Lower saddle height to a workable level and work on hamstring flexibility with a view to progressing to a higher saddle height.

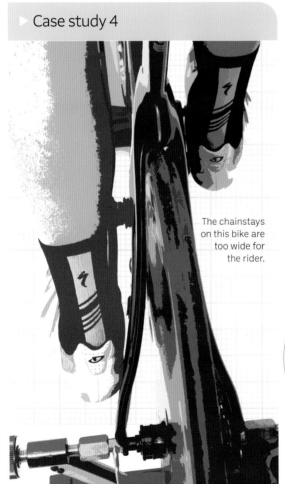

▶ Case study 4

The chainstays on this bike are too wide for the rider.

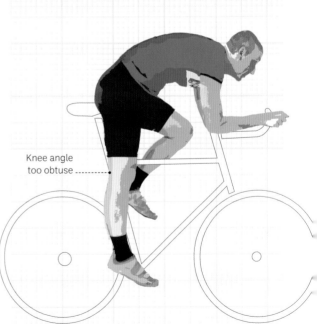

▶ Case study 5

This rider, in trying to set up for time trialling, has put his saddle too high. Note the extended knee at bottom dead centre.

Knee angle too obtuse

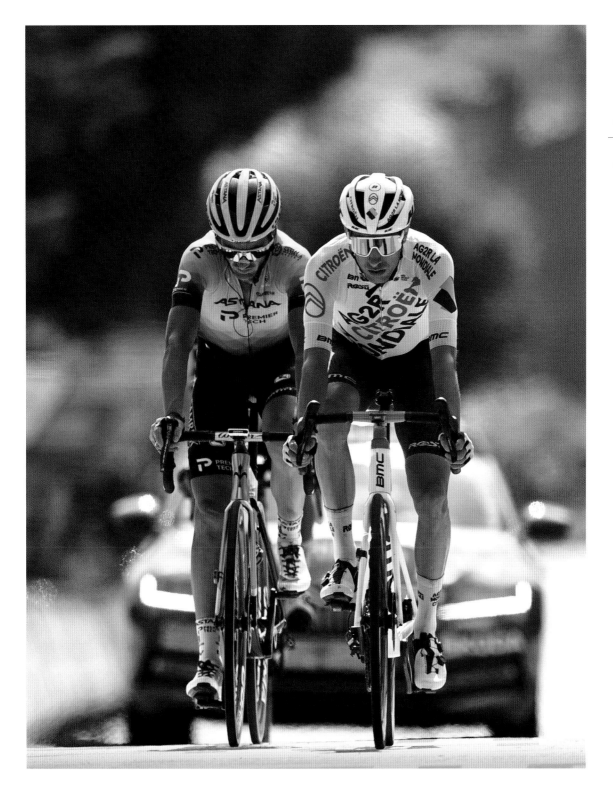

Case study 6

A 45-year-old convert to cycling has been given a bike. She has taken time to set her position up and has set the stem height up to 90mm. All seems fine, except that no matter what she does she spends all her time on the tops and feels the handling is washy around corners.

It's an important question I ask people in pre-bike fit interviews: where do you spend the majority of your time – hoods, drops or tops? If it's the tops it is almost certain your reach set-up is too long and you're bringing your hands to the tops to effectively shorten the reach.

Solution: If the saddle setback is optimal and the stem is already at its shortest safe level, then the bike is most probably too long in the top tube and a frame with a shorter top tube size is required.

Case study 7

A mid-20s rider recently had a crash and fell heavily on his right side and buttock. He returned after the bruising and pain had settled, but ever since has felt twisted on the bike. Subsequently he has felt knee pain on the right side, which has never happened before. It's likely the crash affected the ability of the glutes on his right side to work, which initially led to asymmetrical pelvic alignment that has stuck with him. The twisted pelvis has left him with a functional LLD (see pages 129–131) triggering knee pain, as his set-up does not account for this.

Solution: See a health professional with the skill set to realign the pelvis and reawaken the glute on the right-hand side. In the meantime, address soft tissue changes in the right knee through the use of foam rollers, massage and stretching.

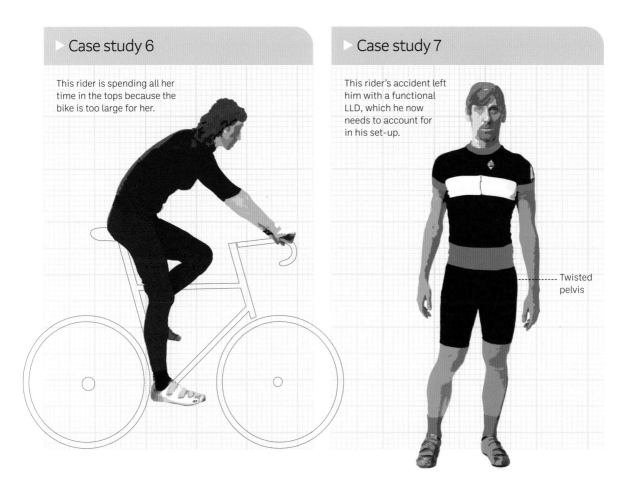

▶ Case study 6

This rider is spending all her time in the tops because the bike is too large for her.

▶ Case study 7

This rider's accident left him with a functional LLD, which he now needs to account for in his set-up.

Twisted pelvis

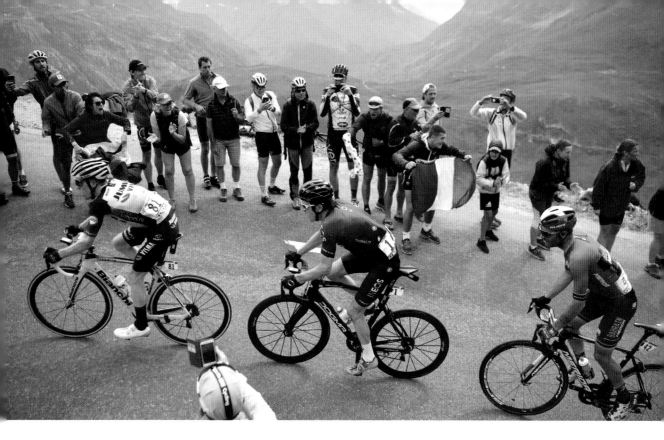

Case study 8

A rider has recently elected to change pedals and shoes, and quickly develops knee pain on both sides, but one more than the other. Further adjustment has led to the pain moving around, rather than going away.

Solution: Changing two contact points at once can be risky. The rider would be well advised to go back to her original set-up, if she still has it, to allow the issue to settle. If it does then we know the change was not just coincidence. She should then change her pedal or her shoe (but not both at once). It may be that this sequential approach allows the rider to transition or that one aspect of the new set-up needs changing.

Case study 9

A rider has been to France for the first time and climbed some of the iconic mountain ascents. Previously the longest he had climbed for was 30 minutes. He developed mild back pain and a sore Achilles tendon on his right side (he knows his right leg is longer than his left).

Mountain climbs can take over two hours for riders at this level – a 300 per cent increase in activity for this rider. In sustained climbing we shuffle back in the saddle, increasing lumbar spine flexion, which can cause aching and pain. We also tend to drop our heels at the bottom of the pedal stroke in sustained climbing, which has caused an acute Achilles tendon issue in the longer leg.

Solution: Seek appropriate care for Achilles tendon and back pain if they persist. Move right cleat rearwards temporarily to help overcome the Achilles tendon issue. Next time, build up longer sustained hill climbing before tackling such a big increase in loading.

Case study 10

A 45-year-old male cyclist who, having ridden a seven-day gravel stage race in South Africa, developed on his return an infection on his perineum that required draining at his local minor injuries unit and treatment with antibiotics. Several months later, following an evening track league, he had a re-occurrence of the infection which cost him more time off the bike, another

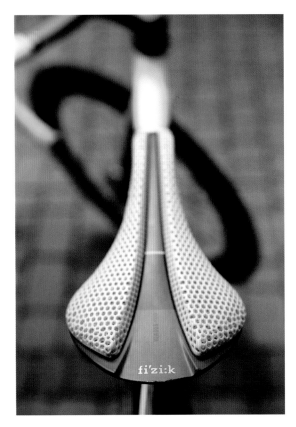

painful trip to minor injuries and involved a further course of antibiotics.

He came to me to see if there were any fit issues that might be contributing to the infections. At the fit, I noticed wear on one side of his chamois of the skin suit he'd been wearing for track league, on one side of his saddle and, on a saddle pressure scan, there was a definite imbalance. Closer inspection of his saddle revealed that one of the rails had begun to collapse and this had thrown his weight distribution off. When we swapped a new saddle in, the scan was even.

He also informed me that on the evening he had noticed soreness on one side and had had to drive home without showering due to an emergency at home. We also examined his training log and noticed that both infections followed periods of high training load.

My suspicion is that the collapsing saddle caused an abrasion that allowed bacteria in and a combination of that, a 45-minute drive in a sweaty skin suit and a lower immune response due to training load led to the second infection.

Solution: A new saddle, a new skin suit and a more thorough approach to checking kit! Once you've had a serious infection, the void that is left will always be more prone to subsequent ones. We put in place a meticulous saddle hygiene routine to combat this. Finally, working with his coach, we looked at how to avoid such a high chronic training load and to incorporate more recovery.

The growing rider

The budding child cyclist presents a constant bike fitting challenge, leading to questions I'm asked all the time: how do I know when to change my child's bike? How do I get him or her to fit properly so that I'm not buying a new bike every six months?

Children grow at different times and different speeds, so there is no one rule that fits all. It is important to accommodate their body on the bike so that they enjoy the experience and are safe. For some (most frequently in the early teens) it is important that they perform to the best of their ability as well. So how do we achieve this?

It's worth remembering that when we are young, we are generally more supple and behave more like macro-absorbers. That means a child can adapt to greater change than an adult and can do so more quickly. Of course, even within the range of children there are more and less adaptable individuals. It's also worth mentioning that a lot of children's bikes are designed in a relaxed fashion to accommodate large changes in size. For instance, there isn't much stack or reach at the front end, so that the handlebars can be reached from more saddle-height positions.

With your budding child cyclist two things are key – measuring them and their bike constantly. By doing this you will be able to spot growth spurts and know when the bike needs adjusting or changing. In children, the key fit parameters on the bike would be knee angle, hip angle and torso angle. A cheap large goniometer will help you establish these angles via the methods described on pages 44–45. The bike itself should be monitored using a tape measure for saddle height, stem length, steerer tube stack, and reach.

Assuming the start position is optimal, the knee and hip joint angles will change as your child grows – they close as the saddle becomes too low (knee extension lessens, hip flex decreases). Adjust the saddle height accordingly to restore the knee and hip joint angles and then the reach (stem length, stack height) to keep the torso angle constant. Once there is excessive seat post showing, or the stem is at 140mm or stack height is 60mm or more, it might be time to consider changing the frame for a larger one as the fit coordinates have run out of room to move and accommodate your child. Crank length is less susceptible to change, but will have to change eventually – every two bike size changes in general.

For this reason, don't spend lots of money on bike frames with kids. At a younger age they are more interested in appearances, so invest in the paint job if anything. Yes, very cheap children's bikes can be heavy and affect enjoyment levels through poor handling, but one could argue it actually improves the child's reactivity. Most kids' racing or road bikes are light enough these days.

I think if you use the concept of the fit window for children you get the best value possible out of the frames and bikes you buy. Establish the above measurements and aim to invest in a bike that has your child at the very bottom of the fit window in terms of saddle height, stem length and stack height. That way they can grow through the fit window and you can adjust the relevant parts as they do.

Of course, sometimes our different body parts grow at different rates. Most of us grow in proportion, but for those who don't the challenge of bike fit is again greater – getting the fit window nailed and starting with the most room to manoeuvre has added importance here.

In terms of how much time a growing child should spend on the bike and at what age, this really isn't my field of expertise. I know with the growth in interest in cycling there is an increased pressure these days at the first talent ID points, for example with British Cycling at Talent and Olympic Development Programme levels.

I would exercise caution in channelling any child's focus to one sport too early, however. The overuse injuries seen in football academies are linked closely to playing competitively too much at too young an age. Keeping a broad range of sports in a child's life to a later age – say 13 or 14 – gives them exposure to a wide variety of movement patterns and challenges physically. This may rob them of specificity in their training, but in my opinion it rewards them later by giving them a wider base of skill application to call on later in life. Remember, children are neuromuscular sponges – the rate at which they learn skills and grow neural pathways to execute them is amazing.

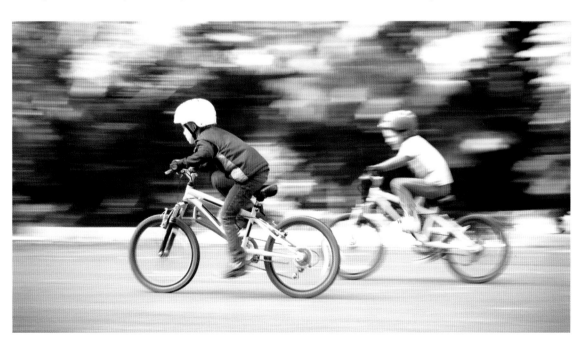

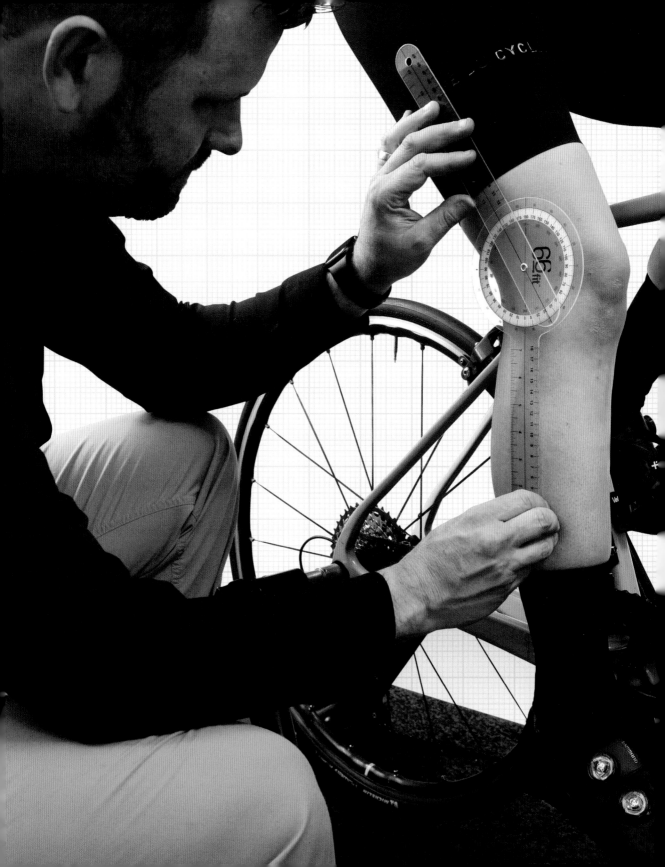

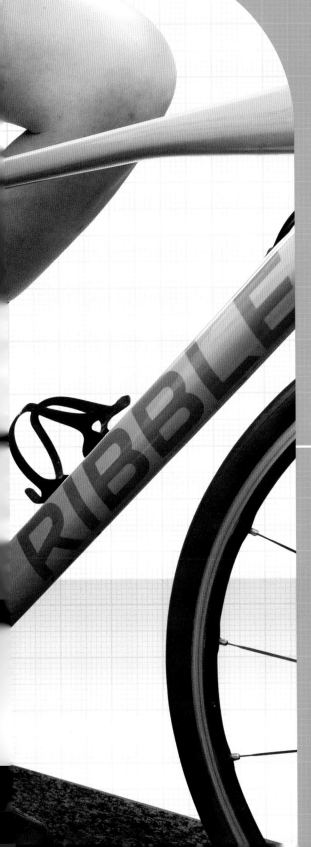

10

Recording your position

Recording your position

Once you have established your optional bike position and are happy with it, make sure you record it! Bike fit is one thing, but trying to replicate your position from bike to bike is another challenge and, unless you have some recorded measurements that you're confident in, it'll always be a struggle.

'm lucky in my studio that I have the Retül Zin tool which creates a digital map of a rider's set-up, which I can then apply to their different bikes quickly and easily. However, with some simple and affordable tools, following the tips below and recording your measurements in the table at the end of this section, you can easily do this for yourself.

Here I have described some easy-to-replicate methods of recording the key parameters that ensure comfort and injury-free riding. Remember, as long as you measure the same way each time from the same reference points, it doesn't matter if your method is different to this. As long as your method is repeatable and consistent, it will work.

Essentials for DIY position recording

▶ Tape measure
▶ Marker pen
▶ Electrical tape
▶ 1m spirit level
▶ Small digital spirit level
▶ A friend to help out can be really useful!

Also remember, there is no one ideal position, just your bike fit window. Employing these techniques and applying your recorded measurements to each bike should see you into that window from which you can then make the small changes that different disciplines, goals, frame geometries and your own evolution as a cyclist demand.

▶ Retül Zin tool

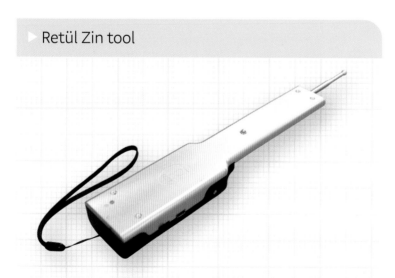

Five essential measurements

▶ Saddle height

On the non-drive side, put your tape measure on the mark in the middle of the bottom bracket.

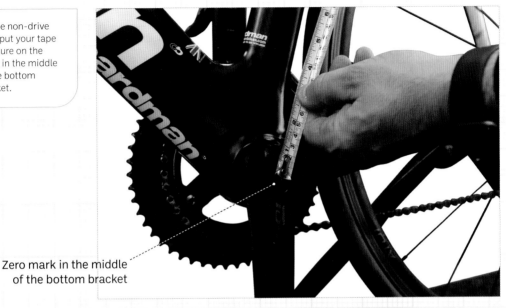

Zero mark in the middle of the bottom bracket

Take the tape measure to a designated place on the saddle (half-way back or 10cm from the front work well and you'll often see white marks on pros' saddles where this has been marked).

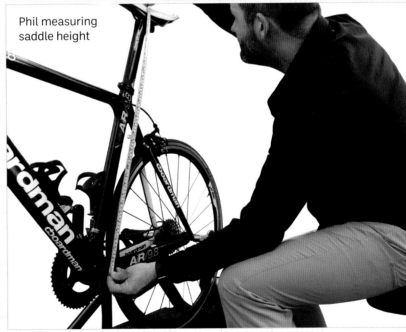

Phil measuring saddle height

▶ Saddle setback

Using a 1m spirit level, place it vertically, so it's in line with the middle of the bottom bracket. Ensure the level is just that – level!

Then use a tape measure to measure the distance from the level to the nose of the saddle.

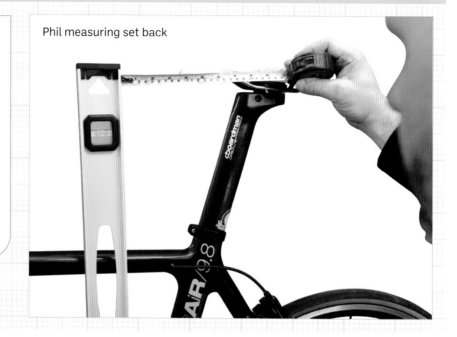

Phil measuring set back

▶ Saddle angle

Use your 1m spirit level between the two wheel skewers to ensure the bike is level.

Then place a small digital spirit level on the saddle.

Where you place the spirit level is important as some saddles are quite long, rise up at the back or have cut-outs, so you are looking for a flat section.

Aside from it being flat, it really doesn't matter exactly where you place the level as long as you measure the same way every time, but I prefer to measure from the middle to the front of a saddle, as that's where saddles tend to be flatter and where most of the riders I work with tend to sit.

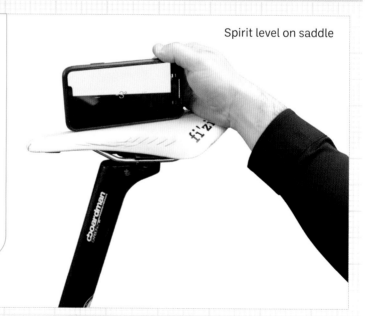

Spirit level on saddle

▶ Reach

This is contact point reach, not frame reach, which you'll find on geometry charts.

This is measured from the front tip of the saddle to the top of the hoods on your bars.

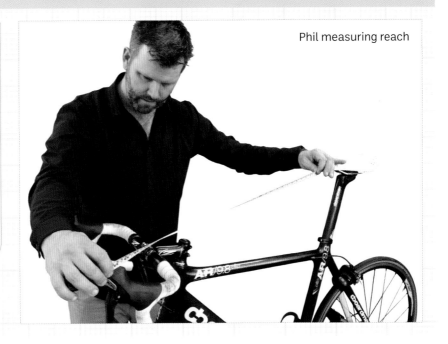

Phil measuring reach

▶ Drop

Again this is contact point drop.

Use the 1m spirit level, rest it on the saddle and extend it forward to the correct level.

Use a tape measure to measure the drop from the level at the front to the handlebars.

This measurement is much easier with a helping hand from a friend.

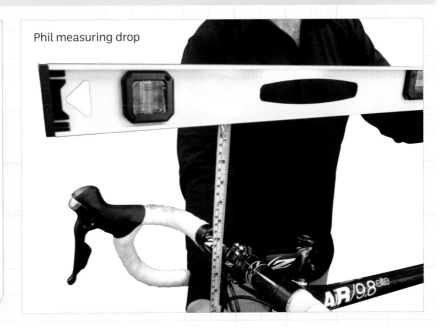

Phil measuring drop

Top tips for replicating your position

▶ Use electrical tape on your seat post to mark your height as this will make it really obvious to see if it has slipped or, if you have to remove your seat post, really easy to drop back into the correct position.

▶ Use a marker pen to mark where your saddle rail clamps are as, like the seat post, these are prone to slipping.

▶ Use a marker pen on the stem and corresponding point on your bars. You'll know, as long as these are lined up, that your bars are correctly rotated and haven't shifted.

▶ Use a marker pen to make a mark on your saddle where you always measure saddle height to.

▶ Photograph your cleat position or use a marker pen to trace around the outside of your cleats (don't rely on the printed lines on the soles of cycling shoes as these are often out).

Other things to note down

▶ Crank length
▶ Saddle width
▶ Saddle length
▶ Handlebar width
▶ Stem length
▶ Number of spacers underneath stem

If you know all the above you can confidently transfer your position from bike to bike.

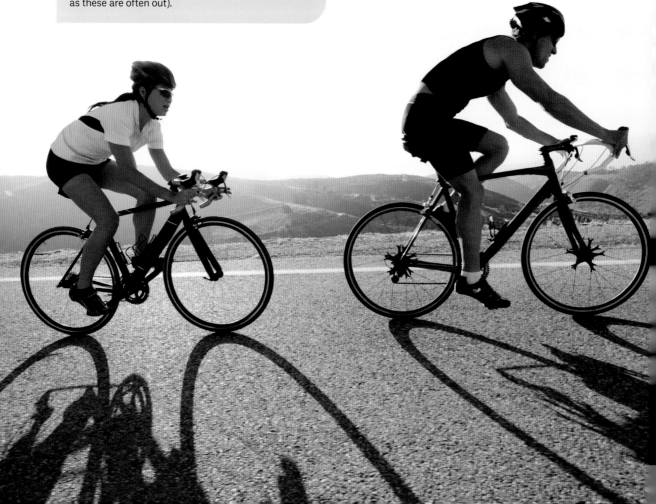

	MEASUREMENT	NOTES
Saddle height		
Saddle setback		
Saddle angle		
Reach		
Drop		
Crank length		
Saddle width		
Saddle length		
Handlebar width		
Stem length		
Number of spacers underneath stem		

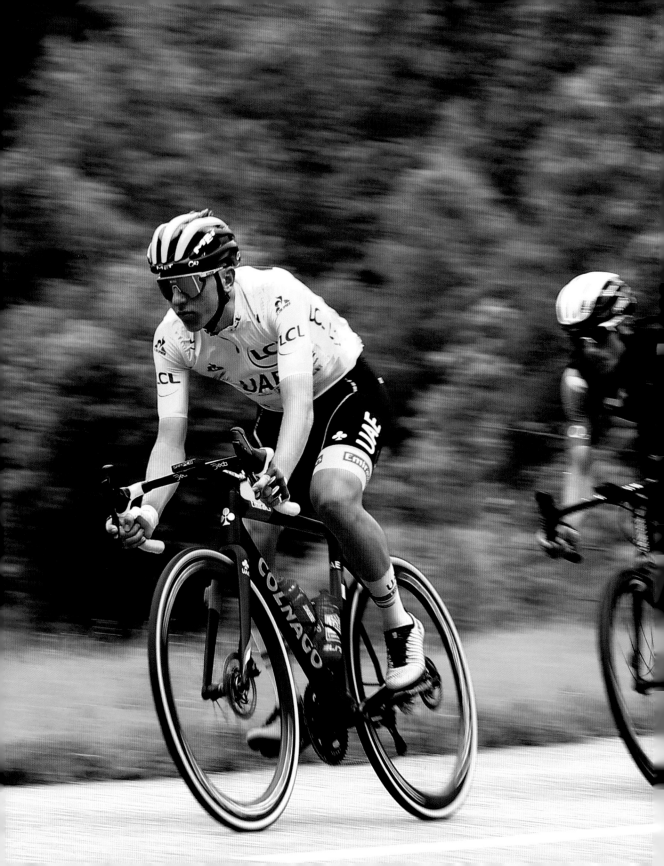

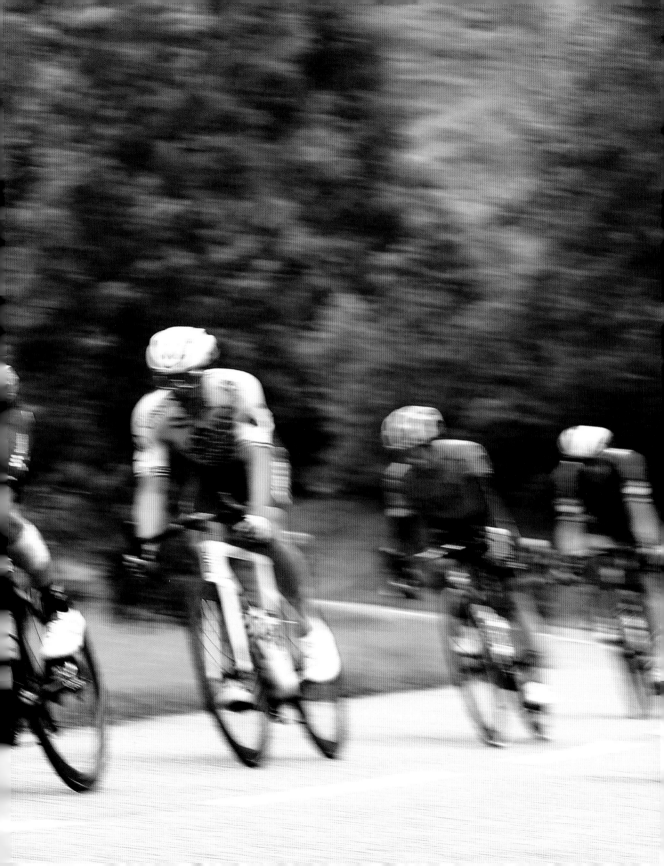

Glossary

accommodative fit – a bike fit that accommodates a person's inflexibilities or issues – the bike comes to the body – not the other way around.

attenuation – absorption or smoothing out of noise. In cycling it's the absorption by the body, and the bike, of the vibration and forces created from the road.

bi-articular muscle – a muscle that crosses two joints in the body and can therefore perform two actions. This is rare. The vast majority of muscles are uni-articular.

BDC – bottom dead centre – referring to the position of the pedal when it is at 6 o'clock or the very bottom of its path.

coefficient of friction – a single number generated from an equation to express the amount of friction acting on – in cycling – the rider and bike.

concentric – a muscle contraction where the muscle shortens, e.g. lifting a tin with your arm to your shoulder – the bicep muscle concentrically shortens.

CONI – the Italian National Olympic Committee (Comitato Olimpico Nazionale Italiano).

coronal plane – see 'frontal plane'.

cortisone – a type of steroid used to control inflammation.

crank arm – the arm that connects the pedal to the chainring and bike.

chainring – the front ring of mounted circular teeth that propels the chain, and bike, forwards.

drops – the loop of handlebar that drops down and back around.

dynamic fit – a bike fit that involves data capture while the rider is the dynamic act of cycling.

eccentrics – a muscle contraction where the muscle lengthens but is still contracting, e.g. slowly lowering a tin from your shoulder to your side – the bicep slowly lengthens – an eccentric contraction.

EMG (electromyography) – electrodes placed on the skin record the electrical activity beneath produced as muscles contract.

evertor – a muscle in lower leg that everts the foot, i.e. moves it towards the outside of the leg.

fascia – connective tissue that overlays muscles and tendons.

femur – the thigh bone.

fit window – the range – for example of saddle height – within which someone can be considered in a good position.

float – the term given to the free movement allowed while the cleats are attached to a clipless or fixed pedal system.

frontal plane – also known as the coronal plane, this is the vertical plane that divides the body into ventral (front) and dorsal (back) sections. It is one of the planes of the body used to describe the location of body parts in relation to each other, see illustration below.

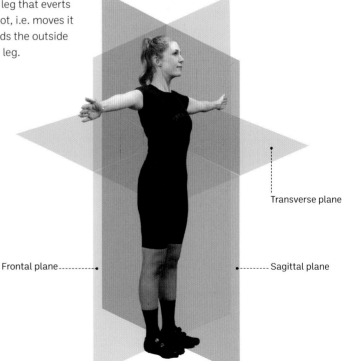

Transverse plane

Frontal plane

Sagittal plane

glutei – the plural of 'gluteus' – a term used to describe all three of the gluteal muscles that form the buttock.

goniometer – a large-arm protractor used for measuring joint angles.

invertor – a muscle of the lower leg that inverts the foot, i.e. turns it inwards.

irregular loading – where a joint or tissue bears weight that it is not designed to cope with or withstand.

isometrics – an isometric contraction is one where the muscle is contracting or working but remains stationary, e.g. holding a tin with your arm in mid-air – the bicep works isometrically to keep it there.

joint angles – the angle formed between two limbs when they meet at a joint, such as at the knee, hip or elbow.

kinetic chain – the chain of limbs, muscles and joints involved in a movement (kinesis).

KOPS – knee over pedal spindle.

neutral fit – a bike fit that places someone in a neutral or safe position, i.e. well within acceptable ranges.

patella – a sesamoid bone sitting in the middle of the quadriceps tendon – also known as the knee cap.

peloton – the name given to the large group of riders that forms in a road race.

plumb bob – a weight attached to a piece of string to aid in finding perfectly vertical positioning, for instance in setting up KOPS.

pronation – movement of the foot and ankle that results in the flattening of the arch of the foot.

pursuiting – the sport in which a rider (or team of riders) pursues another rider (or team) around a track or velodrome.

quadriceps – the group of four muscles on the front of the thigh that help extend or straighten the knee.

rectus femoris – the large bi-articular quadriceps muscle.

sagittal plane – a vertical plane which passes from ventral (front) to dorsal (rear) dividing the body into right and left halves (see illustration).

static fit – a bike fit that takes place with the rider static on the bike, i.e. not cycling.

supination – movement of the foot and ankle that results in arching of the foot.

TDC – top dead centre – referring to the position of the pedal when it is at the 12 o'clock or very top position of its path.

toggling – excessive movement side to side at the pedal cleat engagement due to worn out cleats.

torque – the amount of 'turning force' rotating an object about an axis.

torque chain – a description of the leg muscles involved in the production of torque in cycling.

transverse plane – an imaginary plane that divides the body into superior (upper) and inferior (lower) parts. It is perpendicular to the coronal and sagittal planes (see illustration on the facing page).

valgus – Latin for 'towards the midline' – knock-kneed people have valgus knees. In cycling and bike fitting 'forefoot valgus' relates to the foot being tilted so that the little toe is higher than the big toe, which a shim that cants the foot the opposite way can compensate for.

varus – Latin term for 'away from the midline' – people with splayed-apart knees have varus knee posture. In cycling and bike fitting 'forefoot varus' relates to the foot being tilted so that the big toe is higher than the little toe, which a shim that cants the foot the opposite way can compensate for.

ventilation – the act of breathing – filling and emptying the lungs of air.

UCI – Union Cycliste International – the governing body of world cycling.

Recommended reading and useful websites

A. Baker, *Bike Fit* (4th edn, Argo Publishing/Arnie Baker Cycling, 2009), ebook available from arniebakercycling.com

A. Pruitt, *Andy Pruitt's Complete Medical Guide for Cyclists* (Velopress, 2006)

Bisi M, Ceccarelli M, Riva F, Stagni R. Biomechanical and metabolic responses to seat-tube angle variation during cycling in tri-athletes. *J Electromyog Kinesiol*. 2012;22:845–851. [PubMed][Google Scholar]

Luca De, The C. use of surface electromyography in biomechanics. *J Appl Biomech*. 1997;13:135–163. [Google Scholar]

Dorel S, Couturier A, Hug F. Influence of different racing positions on mechanical and electromyographic patterns during pedaling. *Scand J Med Sci Sports*. 2009;19:44–54. [PubMed][Google Scholar]

Garside I, Doran D. Effects of bicycle frame ergonomics on triathlon 10-km running performance. *J Sports Sci*. 2000;18:825–833. [PubMed] [Google Scholar]

M. Gaskin, *Cycling Science: How Rider and Machine Work Together* (Frances Lincoln, 2013)

Gregor R, Conconi F, Broker J. Biomechanics of road cycling. In: Gregor R, Conconi F, editors. *Road Cycling*. Oxford: Blackwell Science; 2000. pp. 18–39. [Google Scholar]

Hausswirth C, Vallier J, Lehenaff D, Brisswalter J, Smith D, Millet G, Dreano P. Effect of two drafting modalities in cycling on running performance. *Med Sci Sports Exerc*. 2001;33:485–492. [PubMed][Google Scholar]

Heil D, Wilcox A, Quinn C. Cardiorespiratory responses to seat-tube angle variation during steady-state cycling. *Med Sci Sports Exerc*. 1995;27:730–735. [PubMed] [Google Scholar]

Hermens H, Freriks B, Disselhorst-Klug C, Rau G. Development of recommendations for SEMG sensors and sensor placement procedures. *J Electromyog Kinesiol*. 2000;10:361–374. [PubMed][Google Scholar]

Herzog W, Guimaraes A, Anton M, Carter-Erdman K. Moment-length relations of rectus femoris muscles of speed skaters/cyclists and runners. *Med Sci Sports Exerc*. 1991;23:1289–1296. [PubMed][Google Scholar]

J. Hopker and S. Jobson, *Performance Cycling: The Science of Success* (Bloomsbury 2012)

Hug F, Dorel S. Electromyographic analysis of pedaling: A review. *J Electromyog Kinesiol*. 2009; 19:182–189. [PubMed][Google Scholar]

Jeukendrup A, Craig N, Hawley J. The bioenergetics of World Class Cycling. *J Sci Med Sport*. 2000;3:414–433. [PubMed][Google Scholar]

Jorge M, Hull M. Analysis of EMG measurements during bicycle pedaling. *J Biomech*. 1986;19:683–694. [PubMed][Google Scholar]

LaFortune M, Cavanagh P, Valiant G, Burke E. A study of the riding mechanics of elite cyclists. *Med Sci Sports Exerc*. 1983;15:113. [Google Scholar]

Mahony N, Donne B, O'Brien M. A comparison of physiological responses to rowing on friction-loaded and air-braked ergometers. *J Sports Sci*. 1999; 17:143–149. [PubMed][Google Scholar]

Mujika I, Padilla S. Physiological and performance characteristics of male professional road cyclists. *Sports Med*. 2001;31:479–487. [PubMed][Google Scholar]

Price D, Donne B. Effect of variation in seat tube angle at different seat heights on sub-maximal cycling performance in man. *J Sports Sci*. 1997;15:395–402. [PubMed][Google Scholar]

Raasch C, Zajac F, Ma B, Levine W. Muscle coordination of maximum speed pedaling. *J Biomech*. 1997;30:595–602. [PubMed][Google Scholar]

Rankin J, Neptune R. The influence of seat configuration on maximal average crank power during pedaling: A simulation study. *J Appl Biomech*. 2010;26:493–500. [PubMed][Google Scholar]

Reiser R, Peterson M, Broker J. Influence of hip orientation on Wingate power output and cycling technique. *J Strength Cond Res*. 2002;16:556–560. [PubMed][Google Scholar]

Bibliography

Ricard M, Hills-Meyer P, Miller M, Michael T. The effects of bicycle frame geometry on muscle activation and power during a Wingate anaerobic test. *J Sports Sci Med.* 2006;5:25–32. [PMC free article][PubMed][Google Scholar]

Ryan M, Gregor R. EMG profiles of lower extremity muscles during cycling at constant workload and cadence. *J Electromyog Kinesiol.* 1992;2:69–80. [PubMed][Google Scholar]

Savelberg H, van de Port I, Willems P. Body configuration in cycling affects muscle recruitment and movement pattern. *J Appl Biomech.* 2003;19:310–324. [Google Scholar]

Silder A, Gleason K, Thelen D. Influence of bicycle seat tube angle and hand position on lower extremity kinematics and neuromuscular control: Implications for triathlon running performance. *J Appl Biomech.* 2011;27:297–305. [PubMed][Google Scholar]

Winter D, Yack H. EMG profiles during normal human walking: Stride-to-stride and inter-subject variability. *Electroencephalog Clin Neurophysiol.* 1987;67:402–411. [PubMed][Google Scholar]

Websites

retul.com
cyclefit.com
bikefit.com
slowtwitch.com

Anderson. J. and Sockler, J. (1990) 'Effects of orthoses on selected physiological parameters in cycling', *Sports Medicine*, 80(3): 161–5.

Ashe, M. C., Scroop, G. C., Frisken, P. I., Amery, C. A, Wilkins, M. A and Khan, K. M. (2003) 'Body position affects performance in untrained cyclists', *British Journal of Sports Medicine*, 37(5): 441–4.

Barratt, P. R., Korff, T., Elmer, S. J. and Martin, J. C. (2011) 'Effect of crank length on joint-specific power during maximal cycling', *Medicine and Science in Sports and Exercise*, 43(9): 1689–97.

Bini, R. (2012) 'Patellofemoral and tibiofemoral joint forces in cyclists and triathletes: Effects of saddle height', *Journal of Science of Cycling*, 1(1): 9–14 .

Böhm, H., Siebert, S. and Walsh, M. (2008) 'Effects of short-term training using SmartCranks on cycle work distribution and power output during cycling', *European Journal of Applied Physiology*, 103: 225–32

Braeckevelt, I. J., De Bock, I. J., Schuermans, J., Verstockt, S., Witvrouw, E., & Dierckx, J. (2019). The Need for Data-Driven Bike Fitting: Data Study of Subjective Expert Fitting. In: 7th International conference on Sport Sciences Research and Technology (icSports 2019) (pp. 181–189). SCITEPRESS (Science and and Technology Publications).

Broker, J. P. and Gregor, R. J. (1993) 'Mechanical energy management in cycling: Hamstrings and gastrocnemius intercompensate to balance system energy', Department of Physiological Science, University of California, Los Angeles.

Burnett, A., Cornelius, M., Dankaerts, W. and O'Sullivan, P. (2004) 'Spinal kinematics and trunk muscle activity in cyclists: A comparison between healthy controls and non-specific chronic low back pain subjects: A pilot investigation', *Manual Therapy*, 9(4): 211–19.

Clarsen, B., Krosshaug, T. and Bahr, R. (2010) 'Overuse injuries in professional road cyclists', *American Journal of Sports Medicine*, 38(12): 2494–501.

Davids, K., Glazier, P. and Ara, D. (2003) 'Movement systems as dynamical systems: The functional role of variability and its implications for sports medicine', *Sports Medicine*, 33(4): 245–60.

Ellis, R., Hing, W. and Reid, D. (2007) 'Iliotibial band friction syndrome: A systematic review', *Manual Therapy*, 12: 200–8.

Elmer, S. J., Barratt, P. R., Korff, T. and Martin, J. C. (2011) 'Joint-specific power production during submaximal and maximal cycling', *Medicine and Science in Sports and Exercise*, 43(10): 1940-7.

Ericson, M. and Niesell, R. (1986) 'Tibiofemoral joint forces during ergometer cycling', *American Journal of Sports Medicine*, 14(4): 285–90.

Ericson, M., Ekholm, J., Svensson, O. and Nisell, R. (1985) 'The forces of ankle joint structures during ergometer cycling', Foot Ankle, 6(3): 135–42.

Ericson, M., Niesell, R., Arborelius, U. and Ekholm, J. (1985) 'Muscle activity during ergometer cycling', *Scandinavian Journal of Rehabilitation Medicine*, 17:53–61.

Farrell, K., Reisinger, K. and Tillman, M. (2003) 'Force and repetition in cycling: Possible implications for iliotibial band friction syndrome', Knee, 10(1):103–9.

Ferrer-Roca, V., Roig, A., Galilea, P., & García-López, J. (2012). Influence of saddle height on lower limb kinematics in well-trained cyclists: static vs. dynamic evaluation in bike fitting. The Journal of Strength & Conditioning Research, 26(11), 3025-3029. Doi: 10.1519/JSC.0b013e318245c09d.

Francis, P. (1986) 'Injury prevention for cyclists: A biomechanical approach', in E. R. Burke (ed.), *Science of Cycling* (Champaign, IL: Human Kinetics), pp. 145–84.

Fredericson, M., Cookingham, C., Chaudhari, A., Dowdell, B., Oestreicher, N. and Sahrmann, S. (2000) 'Hip abductor weakness in distance runners with iliotibial band syndrome', *Clinical Journal of Sport Medicine*, 10: 169–75.

Fulkerson, J. and Gossling, H. (1980) 'Anatomy of the knee joint lateral retinaculum', *Clinical Orthopaedics and Related Research*, 53: 183–8.

Fulkerson, J. and Hungerford, D. (1990) *Disorders of the Patellofemoral Joint* (Baltimore, MD, Williams and Wilkins).

Gregor, R., Cavanagh, P. and Lafortune, M. (1985) 'Knee flexor moments during propulsion in cycling: A creative solution to Lombard's paradox', *Journal of Biomechanics*, 18(5): 307–16.

Herbert, L. (1994) 'Patellofemoral pain syndrome: The possible role of an inadequate neuromuscular mechanism', *Clinical Biomechanics*, 9(2): 93–7.

Holmes, J. C., Pruitt, A. L. and Whalen, N. J. (1991) 'Cycling knee injuries: Common mistakes that cause injuries and how to avoid them', *Cycling Science*, 3(2): 11–15.

Holmes, J. C., Pruitt, A. L. and Whalen, N. J. (1993) 'Iliotibial band syndrome in cyclists', *American Journal of Sports Medicine*, 21(3): 419–24.

Holmes, J. C., Pruitt, A. L. and Whalen, N. J. (1994) 'Lower extremity overuse in bicycling', *Clinical Sports Medicine*, 13(1): 187–205.

Horton, M. and Hall, T. (1989) 'Quadriceps femoris angle: normal values, and relationships with gender and selected skeletal measures', *Physical Therapy*, 69(11): 897–901.

Hug, F. and Dorel S. (2009) 'Electromyographic analysis of pedaling: A review', *Journal of Electromyography and Kinesiology*, 19(2): 182–98.

Hull, M. L. and Ruby, P. (1996) 'Preventing overuse injuries', in E. R. Burke (ed.), *High-Tech Cycling* (Champaign, IL: Human Kinetics), ch. 11.

Hvid, I., Anderson, B. and Schmidt, H. (1981) 'Chondromalacia patellae: The relation of abnormal joint mechanics', *Acta Orthopaedica*, 52: 661-6.

Hynd, J., Crowle, D., & Stephenson, C. (2014). The influence of hamstring extensibility on preselected saddle height within experienced competitive cyclists. Journal of Science and Cycling, 3(2), 22-22.

Insall, J., Falvo, K. and Wise, D. (1976) 'Chondromalacia patellae: A prospective study', *Journal of Bone Joint Surgery*, 58: 7–8.

Khaund, R. and Flynn, S. (2005) 'Iliotibial band syndrome: A common source of knee pain', *American Family Physician*, 71(8): 1545–50.

Kibler, W., Chandler, T., and Pace, B. (1992) 'Principles of rehabilitation after chronic tendon injuries', *Clinical Journal of Sport Medicine*, 11(3):661–71.

Korff, T., Romer, L. M., Mayhew, I. and Martin, J. C. (2007) 'Effect of pedaling technique on mechanical effectiveness and efficiency in cyclists', *Medicine and Science in Sports and Exercise*, 39(6): 991–5.

Lauterbach, G., Schwellnus, M. and Noakes, T. (1992) 'Biomechanical predictors of overuse knee injuries in cyclists', *Medical Science in Sports and Exercise*, 24(5): S127.

Lavine, R. (2010) 'Iliotibial band friction syndrome', *Current Reviews in Musculoskeletal Medicine*, 3: 18–22.

Lederman, E. (2010) 'The myth of core stability', *Journal of Bodywork and Movement Therapies*, 14(1): 84–98.

Lederman, E. (2011) 'The fall of the postural–structural–biomechanical model in manual and physical therapies: Exemplified by lower back pain', *Journal of Bodywork and Movement Therapies*, 15(2): 131–8.

Martin, J. C. and Brown, N. A. T. (2009) 'Joint-specific power production and fatigue during maximal cycling', *Journal of Biomechanics*, 42: 474–9.

Martin, J. C. and Wagner, B. M. (2002) 'Mechanical energy flow during maximal cycling: Is energy conserved?', in World Congress of Biomechanics 2012.

Martin, J. C., Lamb, S. M. and Brown, N. A. (2002) 'Pedal trajectory alters maximal single-leg cycling power', *Medicine and Science in Sports and Exercise*, 34(8): 1332–6.

Mellion, M. (1991) 'Common cycling injuries: Management and prevention', *Sports Medicine*, 11(1): 52–70.

Nemeth, W. and Sanders, B. (1996) 'The lateral synovial recess of the knee: Anatomy and role in chronic iliotibial band friction syndrome', *Arthroscopy*, 12(5): 574–80.

Neptune, R. R., Kautz, S. A. and Zajac, F. E. (2000) 'Muscle contributions to specific biomechanical functions do not change in forward versus backward pedaling', *Journal of Biomechanics*, 33: 155–164.

Nguyen, A., Boling, M., Levine, B. and Shultz, S. (2009) 'Relationships between lower extremity alignment and the quadriceps angle', *Clinical Journal of Sport Medicine*, 19(3): 201–6.

Olerud, C. and Berg, P. (1984) 'The variation of the quadriceps angle with different positions of the foot', *Clinical Orthopaedics and Related Research*, 79(7): 62–165.

Powers, C., Perry, J., Hsu, A. and Hislop, J. (1997) 'Are patellofemoral pain and quadriceps femoris muscle torque associated with locomotor function?' *Physical Therapy*, 77: 1063-1075.

Price, D. and Donne, B. (1997) 'Effect of variation in seat tube angle at different seat heights on submaximal cycling performance in man', J*ournal of Sports Sciences*, 15(4): 395–402.

Ruby, P. and Hull, M. L. (1993) 'Response of intersegmental knee loads to foot/pedal platform degrees of freedom in cycling', *Journal of Biomechanics*, 26: 1327–40.

Ruby, P., Hull, M., Kirby, K. and Jenkins, D. (1992) 'The effect of lower limb anatomy on knee loads during seated cycling', *Journal of Biomechanics*, 25: 1195–1207.

Salai, M., Brosh, T., Blankstein, A., Oran, A. and Chechik, A. (1999) 'Effect of changing the saddle angle on the incidence of low back pain in recreational bicyclists', *British Journal of Sports Medicine*, 33(6): 398–400.

Sanderson, D. J., Black, A. H. and Montgomery, J. (1994) 'The effect of varus and valgus wedges on coronal plane knee motion during steady-rate cycling', *Clinical Journal of Sport Medicine*, 4: 120-4.

Sanderson, D. J. and Martin, P. E. (1997) 'Lower extremity kinematic and kinetic adaptations in unilateral below-knee amputees during walking', *Gait and Posture*, 6: 126-36.

Sauer, J. L., Potter, J. J., Weisshaar, C. L., Ploeg, H. L., & Thelen, D. G. (2007). Influence of gender, power, and hand position on pelvic motion during seated cycling. Medicine & science in sports & exercise, 39(12), 2204-2211. Doi: 10.1249/mss.0b013e3181568b66.

Schep, G., Bender, M. H., Kaandorp, D., Hammacher, E. and de Vries, W. R. (1999) 'Flow limitations in the iliac arteries in endurance athletes: Current knowledge and directions for the future', *International Journal of Sports Medicine*, 20(7): 421–8.

Silberman, M. R., Webner, D., Collina, S. and Shiple, B. J. (2005) 'Road bicycle fit', *Clinical Journal of Sport Medicine*, 15(4): 271–6.

Tamborindeguy, A. and Bini, R. (2011) 'Does saddle height affect patellofemoral and tibiofemoral forces during bicycling for rehabilitation?', *Journal of Bodywork and Movement Therapies*, 15(2): 186–191.

Too, D. (1994) 'The effect of trunk angle on power production in cycling', *Research Quarterly for Exercise and Sport*, 65(4): 308–15.

Weiss, B. (1985) 'Non-traumatic injuries in amateur long distance bicyclists', *American Journal of Sports Medicine*, 13(3): 187–92.

Wilber, C. A., Holland, G. J., Madison, R. E. and Loy, S. F. (1995) 'An epidemiological analysis of overuse injuries among recreational cyclists', *International Journal of Sports Medicine*, 16(3): 201–6.

Index

Acknowledgements

I would like to acknowledge firstly anyone who has contributed to this book and isn't mentioned shortly – you know who you are and the book is all the better for your input.

Specific thanks go to Nik Cook, Sarah Skipper, Charlotte Croft, Grant Pritchard and as always the unflappable David Luxton.

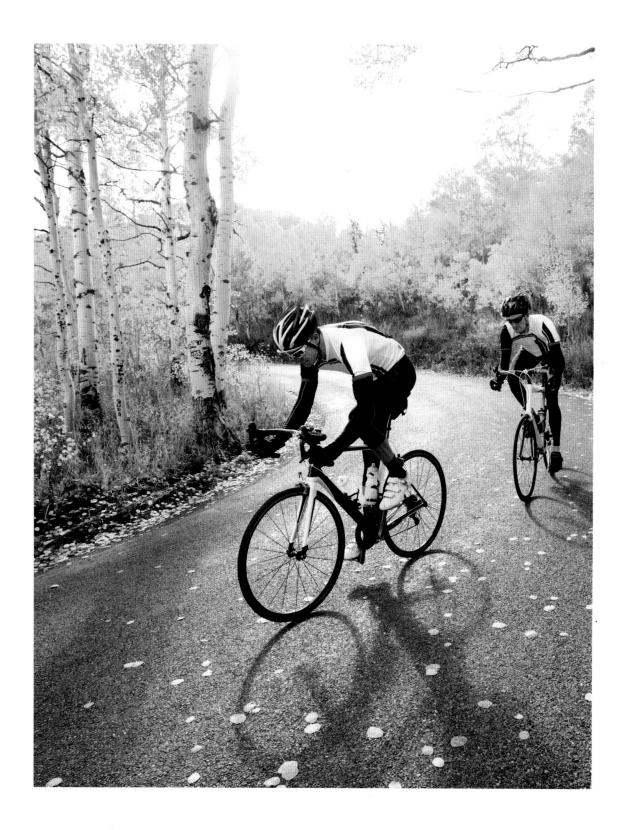